The Politics of Polio in Northern Nigeria

ELISHA P. RENNE

The Politics of Polio
in Northern Nigeria

INDIANA UNIVERSITY PRESS
Bloomington and Indianapolis

This book is a publication of

Indiana University Press
601 North Morton Street
Bloomington, Indiana 47404-3797 USA

www.iupress.indiana.edu

Telephone orders	800-842-6796
Fax orders	812-855-7931
Orders by e-mail	iuporder@indiana.edu

♾ The paper used in this publication meets the minimum requirements
of the American National Standard for Information Sciences—
Permanence of Paper for Printed Library Materials, ANSI Z39.48-1992.

Manufactured in the United States of America

Library of Congress Cataloging-in-Publication Data
Renne, Elisha P.
  The politics of polio in northern Nigeria / Elisha P. Renne.
      p.   ; cm.
  Includes bibliographical references and index.
  ISBN 978-0-253-35515-7 (cloth : alk. paper) — ISBN 978-0-253-22228-2
(pbk. : alk. paper)   1. Poliomyelitis—Nigeria, Northern.   I. Title.
  [DNLM: 1. Poliomyelitis—prevention & control—Nigeria.
2. Health Policy—Nigeria.   3. Immunization—ethics—Nigeria.
4. Poliomyelitis—economics—Nigeria.   WC 556 R414p 2010]
  RA644.P9R46 2010
  362.196'835009669—dc22
                                        2010002427

1   2   3   4   5   15   14   13   12   11   10

For JSS.

Contents

Acknowledgments

In researching and writing this book, I have incurred many debts over the years. Colleagues at Ahmadu Bello University and Nuhu Bamalli Polytechnic—both in Zaria—have, from the beginning, been extraordinarily generous with their time and advice. They include Mairo Bugaje, Sheikh Dan Ladi, Clara Ejembi, Rabiu Mohammed Isah, Salihu Maiwada, Mairo Mandara, Musa Muhammed, S. O. Shittu, Ya'u Tanimu, Dakyes Usman, and A. M. Yakubu, as well as J. B. Familusi of the University of Ibadan, among many others who have helped me in myriad ways. I am also grateful to Osman Alhassan and Samuel Ntewusu for their kind guidance concerning my research in Yendi, Ghana, and to K. O. Antwi Agyei for information about Ghana NIDs. At the University of Michigan, I have benefited from the comments and suggestions of faculty—Stuart Batterman, Kofi Gyan, Sioban Harlan, Marcia Inhorn (now at Yale), Stuart Kirsch, Jerome Nriagu, Maxwell Owusu, Afeworki Paulos (now at Carnegie Mellon), and Holly Peters-Golden—and of the students who worked with me in Zaria City—Roopa Akkineni, Viola Allo Allo, and Kelly Kirby. Funds from the Department of Anthropology, from the Center for Afroamerican and African Studies, and from the Advanced Study Center of the International Institute, University of Michigan, facilitated this study, as did the exceptional assistance of University of Michigan librarians who were able to locate seemingly unobtainable sources. Map librarian Karl Longstreth was particularly helpful, as was Caitlin Couture. In addition, I would like to thank colleagues and friends whom I imposed on for advice, a second reading, and solace—Laura Arntson, Chris Bankole, Sue Bergh, LaRay Denzer, Stephen Kunitz, and Murray Last, as well as the late Philip Shea, as well as Dee Mortensen, Peter Froehlich, and Brian Herrmann at Indiana University Press.

The research on which this book is based would not have been possible without the patient and tolerant cooperation of many people in Zaria, Samaru, Kaduna, Kano, Likoro, and Solanke, as well as Ibadan and Lagos, in Nigeria, and in Accra, Yendi, and Tamale in Ghana, who agreed to be interviewed. Without their frank and detailed explanations, it would have been very difficult to understand, let alone explain, why the Polio Eradication Initiative met the resistance that it did. Above all, I would like to thank His Royal Highness the Emir of Zazzau, Dr. Shehu Idris, CFR, for granting me permission to stay in Zaria City, and the former vice chancellor of Ahmadu Bello University, Professor A. M. Abdullahi, whose kindness over the years has reassured me in this project. Thanks also go to Alhaji Ahamed Muhammed for allowing me to stay in his house in Zaria City since 1994 and to Sani Ibrahim, Umma Yahaya, Malam Mohammed Mohammed, Alhaji Sa'idu Ibrahim Halidu, and Josiah Olubowale for special assistance.

While I can hardly compile an exhaustive list of all those who deserve thanks,

I would like to close by acknowledging the support of Malam Ya'u Tanimu and Hassana Yusuf, who have helped me since the beginning of my stay in Zaria. Together, they helped me to organize research assistance, provided excellent counsel and information, and patiently waited with me when I needed visa extensions. My visits to Hassana's parents' home in Kaduna were always a pleasant respite from what was, at times, a difficult research project. Hassana Yusuf continues to impress me with her willingness to pursue difficult leads and recalcitrant informants as well as to suffer through long and uncomfortable bus and taxi rides without complaint. To her I owe special thanks.

Hannu daya ba ya daukan jinka

The Politics of Polio in Northern Nigeria

1. Introduction: Protesting Polio

Poliomyelitis did not attract medical attention in West Africa until the last 20 years. Because it was considered rare, Gelfand and Miller (1956) recommended that prophylactic polio-vaccination was not necessary in the indigenous population.

—Familusi and Adesina, "Poliomyelitis in Nigeria"

Polio has spread to two more countries in West Africa, further jeopardizing the World Health Organization's goal of wiping out the crippling disease by next year. . . . WHO officials are placing the blame squarely with Nigeria, which is Africa's most populous nation and home of 300 of the new polio cases in 2003, nearly half the world total.

—Altman, "Polio cases in West Africa may thwart W.H.O. plan"

Many aspects of our own contemporary culture might be called premonitory shivers: panicky renderings of unreadable messages about the kind of society we are creating.

—Kuhn, *Soulstealers*

One day in early August 2005 in Zaria City, an anxious father approached me for advice about what he should do for his fifteen-year-old son whose left leg had become paralyzed. I suggested that he take his child to the nearby university teaching hospital, where surely they would be able to diagnose the cause of the problem. I also asked him if perhaps it might be polio, not certain whether he had had his son immunized against the disease. He assured me that he had and that, furthermore, wasn't he too old to contract polio—or Shan Inna, as it is called in Northern Nigeria? I said I wasn't sure but that he should take his son to the hospital as soon as possible.[1]

When I saw him later that week, he said that they had taken an X-ray of the boy's leg at the hospital but were unable to determine the cause of the paralysis. He thought that perhaps it was typhoid fever, but they had dismissed this possibility and said instead that the child must have injured the leg somehow. They then gave the child an injection which seemed to make things worse. He would cry all night because of the pain, and the tablets they gave him did not seem to help.

A few days later, I was leaving the house to visit a retired government official and ran into the man again. This time, he was with his wife and another woman, both dressed in long, dark hijabs. One was carrying the boy, whose left leg dangled limply down her back. When I asked where they were going, the husband explained that they were taking the boy to a traditional healer in Kano to find a cure for his leg. When I stopped by their house a few days later, they had not yet returned.

The following week, when my neighbor returned from Kano with his son, he explained that the *malam* or Muslim teacher to whom they'd taken the boy said that it was a spirit that was causing the problem. He prayed, and within two days after they returned to Zaria there was a darkening near the child's ankle and a boil formed. When he saw the boil, he called the *malam* on his cell phone to ask if he should bring the boy back to Kano. "No, no," the *malam* said, "take him to the teaching hospital for them to lance it and that will be the end of it." He did so, the wound healed, and the boy was able to walk again.

*　*　*

The uncertain cause of this young boy's paralysis and the apparent inability of Western medicine to cure it captures a sense of the confusion and fear which surrounded the international effort to eradicate poliomyelitis in Northern Nigeria. Paralysis of one or more limbs is a characteristic symptom of polio, yet paralysis may have other causes as well. Indeed, the difficulty of conducting laboratory tests to distinguish cases of polio from other cases of acute flaccid paralysis (paralysis in one or more limbs), has been one of the major challenges of its eradication. In *The Politics of Polio in Northern Nigeria,* I examine the Polio Eradication Initiative as it was conducted from 1988 to mid-2009, focusing on the ways that this campaign has been viewed by men and women living in Northern Nigeria, where some, but not all, parents have refused to have their children immunized against the disease. In 2006, Northern Nigeria had the largest number of wild poliovirus cases in the world. Although this number declined substantially in 2007 and then increased in 2008, it has declined again in 2009 (WHO 2009; table 1.1). My aim here is to explain why national and international health workers have encountered resistance to this initiative by situating the eradication campaign within the social, political, and historical context of people's experience of polio in Northern Nigeria. This experience includes the treatment of paralysis during the precolonial period, colonial medical personnel's lack of concern with polio as compared with other infectious diseases, the deterioration of primary health care in Nigeria during the 1990s, the polio immunization boycott in Kano State in 2003–2004, and the recent outbreak of circulating vaccine-derived poliovirus in 2005–2009. I also consider the responses of WHO, UNICEF, CDC, and USAID personnel to these events and to continuing resistance to the Polio Eradication Initiative, particularly health workers' development of the Immunization Plus Days program in 2006, which addressed parents' concerns about malaria and other health problems more relevant to them. In this program, health workers go house-to-house, providing polio vaccines, Vitamin A drops, deworming medicines, and insecticide-treated bednets to protect against malaria-carrying mosquitos. By considering Northern Nigerian parents' belief that government and associated health organizations should provide basic health services, these officials indirectly acknowledged that opposition to the Polio Eradication Initia-

Table 1.1. Cases of Acute Flaccid Paralysis (AFP) and Confirmed Cases of Wild Poliovirus and Circulating Vaccine-Derived Poliovirus, Nigeria, 1999–2009 (as of 11 December 2009)

Year	AFP cases reported	Non-polio AFP rate	AFP cases w/adequate specimens (%)	Total confirmed polio cases	Wild-virus confirmed polio cases	Vaccine-derived confirmed polio cases
1999	1242	0.5	26	981	98	—
2000	979	0.7	36	638	28	—
2001	1937	3.8	67	56	56	—
2002	3010	5.7	84	202	202	—
2003	3318	6.0	91	355	355	—
2004	4814	8.0	91	782	782	—
2005	4836	6.3	85	831	830	1
2006	5175	6.5	88	1143	1122	21
2007	4277	5.9	94	353	285	68
2008	5538	6.6	93	861	799	62
2009	5048	7.1	95	534	386	148

Source: WHO 2009 (http://www.who.int/immunization_monitoring/en/diseases/poliomyelitis/ case_count.cfm, accessed 11 December 2009).

tive reflected, in part, the inadequacy of a universal eradication protocol which failed to take the collapse of primary health care in Nigeria, particularly routine immunization, into account.

However, as Hardon and Blume (2005, 353) have observed, "it is difficult to criticize a vaccine initiative." While many Northern Nigerians saw the benefits of vaccinating their children against polio, some protested against the campaign by refusing to have their children immunized. They were often characterized as misled by Muslim leaders, as deceived by rumors, or as illiterate and irresponsible parents. One might well question the ethics of parents who reject immunization against polio or other infectious diseases for their children. However, those who refused saw their actions as the most ethical ones possible in the face of uncertainty about the safety of the polio vaccine. Like parents in the U.S. who "may prefer to make errors of omission . . . rather than errors of commission" (Fredrickson et al. 2004, 432) and therefore refuse to have their children immunized, some Northern Nigerian parents, because of fears of contaminated vaccines, decided not to have their children immunized (Blume 2006).[2]

While this book focuses on the town of Zaria in Northern Nigeria (map 1.1), I also examine the implementation and reception of the Polio Eradication Initiative in Northeastern Ghana (in chapter 6) in order to provide a comparative perspective that clarifies both the similarities and differences in ways that polio eradication has been experienced in different West African countries. While these two regions share environmental and religious similarities—both are dry

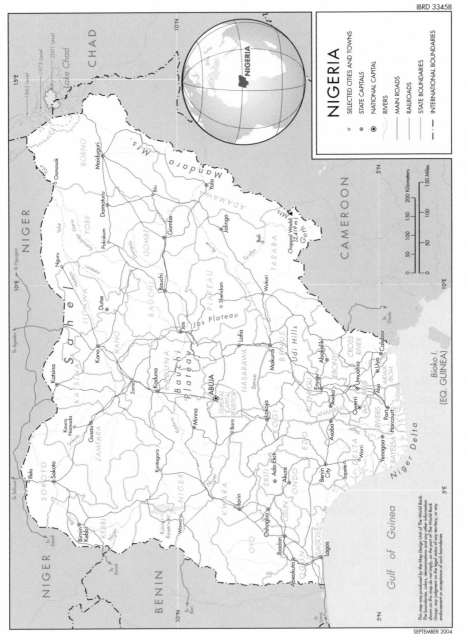

Map 1.1. Map of Nigeria, indicating the locations of Zaria, Kaduna, and Kano. Courtesy of the World Bank.

savannah areas with large Muslim populations—differences in the campaign's implementation reflect their distinctive sociocultural, economic, and political histories as well as differences in their overall levels of immunization and in the continuity of national and health department leadership. The situation in Northern Nigeria has enabled wild poliovirus to spread to Northeastern Ghana (as well as to several other West African countries, including Benin, Burkina Faso, Chad, Mali, Niger, and Togo). In 2008, eight cases in Ghana were attributed to strains of poliovirus originating in Northern Nigeria, which were identified by genomic sequencing techniques.

Poliomyelitis (literally, inflammation of the grey marrow, i.e., of the central nervous system) is caused by a type of enterovirus found throughout the world. Since it is spread mainly through fecal-oral transmission—which can occur when people swallow contaminated water or eat foods which have come into contact with contaminated water or feces—the environmental context strongly influences who contracts polio and at what age. In environments with few or no public sanitation systems, infants often contract asymptomatic cases of polio which result in sufficient antibodies to confer immunity (Paul 1971, 358). In these cases, the poliovirus remains in the alimentary tract, primarily in the small intestine, where the body's immune system produces antibodies that counter the virus, which is subsequently excreted, usually within a period of a few weeks. In rare instances— approximately one in two hundred cases—the virus penetrates the central nervous system, particularly the grey matter of the spinal column, where it causes lesions which, if extensive, affect the motor nerve supply of the muscles, resulting in paralysis (Paul 1971, 2–3). However, as Paul (1971, 365) has noted,

> When poliovirus infection is restricted to the youngest age group (0–4 years) more than 95 percent of such infections are inapparent. On the other hand, when school children and adolescents represent the most susceptible groups, the percentage of inapparent infection falls off progressively with age and far more individuals experience a paralytic attack.

The polio epidemics of twentieth-century America were, ironically, the result of improved standards of public sanitation (Rogers 1992); children were not exposed to the wild poliovirus until they were older, when the disease was more likely to result in paralysis and could be fatal. The massive polio epidemics of the 1940s and 1950s contributed to American parents' initial widespread acceptance of the Salk polio vaccine (Colgrove 2006; Oshinsky 2005). In Nigeria, where public sanitation was (and continues to be) poor, poliomyelitis has never been seen as a major health problem because many acquire immunity through environmental exposure as infants, when polio symptoms are mainly restricted to fevers and only a small fraction of cases result in paralysis.

Thus, in Nigerian parents' experience, paralytic polio was a relatively rare event, and malaria and measles were the major killers of children (Schimmer and Ihekweazu 2006). The focus on polio in the late 1990s led some parents to question why their government and international organizations associated with the West (such as Rotary International, the Gates Foundation, CDC, WHO, and

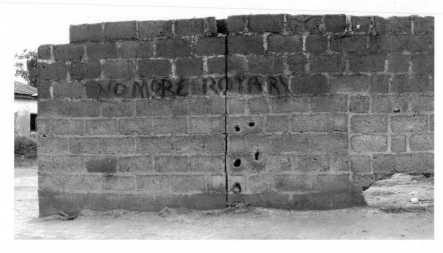

Figure 1.1. Walls often provide a site for the airing of public opinion. This wall, along the main thoroughfare leading to the Emir of Zaria's palace in Zaria City, had the phrase "No More Rotary" painted on it around 2005, a reference to Rotary International's sponsorship of the Polio Eradication Initiative. The words were no longer visible in 2009. Photograph by E. P. Renne, Zaria City, August 2007.

UNICEF) were supporting such a program.[3] For them, the risk of their children being paralyzed by polio did not offset the risks associated with contaminated vaccines, and moreover they distrusted the motives of their government and the international organizations (fig. 1.1). As one farmer living near Zaria explained,

> No, I don't allow the people to do polio vaccination for my children in the house because there is a problem in it, such as that European people want us to reduce our numbers, to stop us from giving birth. And [when] we are looking for medicine in the hospital to give to our children and we can't get it but this one, they are following us to our houses to give it. I don't trust this polio vaccine. (Interview, Samaru, September 2005)[4]

Ideas about the oral polio vaccine and about immunization more generally—which may be seen as protecting healthy individuals against disease or as threatening them with harm—reflect local definitions of a particular disease as well as views on public health, the responsibility of government and the ethics of its initiatives, and the politics of international relations.

Indeed, this intersection and, at times, conflict between the concerns and actions of Northern Nigerian parents and of those acting for national health institutions and international public health organizations represents a particular form of structural inequality (Farmer 1999, 2005). Specifically, immunization campaigns that are organized by those in positions of power and resisted by those with relatively little power exemplify a subversion of dominance, what James Scott (1985) has referred to as "weapons of the weak." These everyday forms of subversion against government programs may take the form of "passive noncompliance, subtle sabotage, evasion, and deception" (Scott 1985, 29; see also Nations and Monte 1996). In Zaria City—the walled section of the larger town of Zaria, which is the center of the old emirate of Zazzau—they took several forms. When health workers came to their houses, parents sometimes denied having children staying with them.[5] Or they would mark the doorways of their houses as the health workers did after their visits, as though vaccinations had already taken place there.[6] Distrust of the West among Muslim Hausa men and women in Northern Nigeria reflects both their apprehension about U.S. and European actions in the Middle East (M. Last 2008) and their disapproval of their own government's supporting international health programs while failing to provide local primary health care (Yahya 2007). Their refusal to participate in the Polio Eradication Initiative represents their way of countering these unequal power relations and of affecting the conduct of the initiative, in which they initially had no say. By protesting the Polio Eradication Initiative, with its initial exclusive focus on polio and failure to address other, more serious child health problems, Northern Nigerian parents were able to obtain—with the implementation of the 2006 Immunization Plus Days—a health intervention that was meaningful for them.

Certainly, not all Northern Nigerian parents have responded to the Polio Eradication Initiative in this way. Those in positions of relative power are less likely to do so. Many, but not all, parents with advanced levels of Western education, for example, have allowed their children to be immunized (M. Muhammed 2003; National Population Commission and ORC Macro 2004;). However, the nature of polio transmission, immunization, and verification makes it difficult to eradicate polio in Nigeria without a continued, concerted effort, even when resistance to polio vaccination is much reduced and overall levels of immunization have improved.

Primary Health Care and the Polio Eradication Initiative in Nigeria

Eradicating polio in Nigeria, i.e., breaking the chain of transmission of the poliomyelitis virus, as evidenced by a lack of new confirmed cases within a given time frame (Yekutiel 1980, 24) and the subsequent certification of a total absence of cases (Miller, Barrett, and Henderson 2006, 1164), would be difficult under any circumstances. Nigeria is the most populous country in sub-Saharan Africa, with a population of 148,093,000 in 2007 (UNICEF 2009). Many live in megacities such as Lagos and Kano, while others live in towns, villages, and hamlets dispersed over a landmass of 356,669 square miles (923,768 sq. km) and connected by a system of roads in varying states of repair.[7] While Nigeria is rich in natural resources (particularly petroleum), political instability and economic inequality have contributed to a lack of continuity in national leadership and development policies as well as to a decline in the country's infrastructure.

This political situation has also contributed to frequent changes in federal health leadership and to the decline of primary health care in Nigeria, which is reflected in community health clinics, often without water or electricity and with a shortage of trained medical staff. Nigeria, until recently, had extremely low rates of general immunization nationally, estimated at 12.9 percent in 2003 (National Population Commission and ORC Macro 2004, 130), although rates have improved, being estimated at 54 percent in 2006 (WHO and UNICEF 2007). Improved provision of vaccines at neighborhood health centers and through Immunization Plus Days has contributed to this change.[8]

However, other logistical problems are also associated with the goal of eradicating polio. The example of the young boy whose leg became paralyzed exemplifies the difficulties of distinguishing poliomyelitis from other causes of acute flaccid paralysis, such as Guillain-Barré syndrome and acute myelopathy associated with various infections (Hull 2004, 698). In order to definitively confirm cases of polio, two stool samples, taken within two weeks of the onset of paralysis, must be analyzed in a laboratory. The challenges of confirming reports of paralyzed infants and young children, getting stool samples, and then transporting them on ice to laboratories in Ibadan, to the south, or Maiduguri, to the northeast, are enormous. Another difficulty is that oral polio vaccine, the type of vaccine used in Nigeria (and throughout Africa), requires three or four doses for complete immunity. Thus, parents may believe that their children have been immunized when in fact they have received only one or two doses and are still susceptible to the disease.[9]

In addition to the difficulties of confirming the presence of the poliovirus and of ensuring that children received the requisite number of doses of polio vaccine, two other problems contributed to misunderstandings and confounded the work of health personnel. In 2007, four children in Kaduna State had confirmed cases of polio, although two had received three doses of the vaccine and one had received four doses (WHO Kaduna 2007b). There are several possible explanations for these children's contracting polio despite having been vaccinated. First, antibodies ingested through their mothers' milk can deactivate the vaccine in breast-fed infants under six months old (Familusi and Adesina 1977, 123). Second, the children may have been suffering from other enteroviral infections at the time the received polio vaccine. Third, the vaccine may have become ineffective as a result of heat or mishandling. Finally, in the absence of record cards, the mothers may have misrepresented the number of doses of vaccine their children had received. Another problem is that the Sabin oral polio vaccine consists of an attenuated virus that, in rare instances, may revert back to its original potency in the environment (Kew et al. 2004). From July 2005 to June 2009, there were 255 confirmed cases of circulating vaccine-derived poliovirus in Northern Nigeria (CDC 2009a). These aspects of oral polio vaccination not only suggest the difficulties health officials faced during the polio campaign but also the difficulties parents faced in weighing the benefits and risks of immunizing their children. When parents have themselves experienced paralytic polio or have children or relatives who have, they may see immunization as a lower risk by comparison.

Those who view paralytic polio as uncommon may see the risk associated with oral polio vaccine as a relatively greater one.

In the case of the young boy with the paralyzed leg with which I opened this chapter, the inability of hospital doctors to diagnose the cause of the boy's paralysis further contributed to the questioning of the value of Western medicine more generally. Since the hospital personnel were unable to provide treatment—indeed, they exacerbated the problem by giving the boy an antibiotic injection in his paralyzed limb—the child's parents sought alternative traditional therapy, which appeared to be successful, additionally undermining the authority of Western biomedicine and its claims to superior knowledge. The distrust raised by the contradictory claims of medical authorities—that they know the best ways to preserve the health of children, yet are sometimes wrong—along with the logistics of immunizing all children under five years of age with three (and optimally four) doses of oral polio vaccine has made the eradication of polio in Northern Nigeria an extremely difficult goal to achieve.

Politics and Polio in Nigeria

Northern Nigeria, one of the four remaining areas in the world where wild poliovirus continues to circulate, has been cited frequently in the Western press as a source of infection for formerly polio-free countries and an obstacle to the global effort to eliminate polio worldwide (Altman 2004; McNeil 2008b). While Northern Nigerian Muslim religious leaders and parents who believed that the oral polio vaccine was contaminated—with HIV-AIDS, infertility drugs, or other substances—have often been blamed for the failure to eradicate wild poliovirus in Nigeria,[10] the political context of the Polio Eradication Initiative has not been adequately examined. Indeed, the politics of polio eradication in Nigeria have been a significant obstacle to eradication efforts. Ferguson (1994) has noted the general tendency of development agencies to overlook political aspects of project proposals. The Polio Eradication Initiative provides yet another example of how politics—at the local, national, and international levels—may undermine even the best of intentions.

In Nigeria, the Polio Eradication Initiative came at a time of tremendous political turmoil, with the death of General Sani Abacha in June 1998, the year-long interim presidency of General Adulsalami Abubakar, and the election in February 1999 of General Olusegun Obasanjo, who was inaugurated in May 1999 (Synge 2001). While President Obasanjo appointed Professor Eyitayo Lambo as the new minister of health, the National Programme on Immunization—a parastatal government body directly responsible to the president, which was set up under the Abacha regime—was left in place.

The fact that Abacha and Abubakar were also Hausa-Fulani Muslims[11] and that Obasanjo was a Yoruba Christian would seem to reinforce the widespread stereotype of Nigeria as divided into a Muslim north and a Christian south. This stereotype, however, is complicated by a number of factors relating to religion, ethnicity, and history, which cross-cut and undermine any such simple dichotomies.

For example, those who identify themselves as of Yoruba ethnicity may also distinguish themselves by geographic areas and linguistic sub-ethnic groups, and they are equally likely to be Christian or Muslim (Eades 1980, 128; M. Last 2007, 607); among Yoruba living in Northern Nigeria there are both Christians and Muslims (Olaniyi 2006). While Christian missionaries during the nineteenth and twentieth centuries were able to convert many Yoruba men and women, many also converted to Islam as a result of the historical influence of the powerful Sokoto Caliphate, which dominated religious and political life in Northern Nigeria in the nineteenth century. I make this point here to emphasize that for many Yoruba, Christians and Muslims alike, monotheistic religions are not a significant divisive factor within Yoruba communities, where specific Yoruba social identities (e.g., family ties and political affiliation) are the critical aspects. If there are religious tensions, they are more likely to exist between those maintaining traditional Yoruba religious practices and followers of the two monotheisms, Christianity and Islam. Regardless of these religious differences, Western education provided by missionaries and colonial government schools was generally viewed as valuable.

However, in Northern Nigeria, Muslim identity is a critical factor for many, although believers are divided among different Islamic sects: Qadiriyya, Tijaniyya, Izala, Shi'a, Sufi, and, more recently, Salafiyya.[12] Class, as reflected in royal or commoner birth and in wealth, and place of origin are also important constituents of identity.[13] Despite these differences, what has been of critical importance in reinforcing a Muslim identity in the North is the Qur'an. Before the coming of British colonial rule in 1903 and the establishment of Western primary schools (boko), there was a network of Islamic schools, some teaching basic rote learning, with students using allo (wooden boards used to write and to memorize passages from the Qur'an), and Islamiyya schools where students are taught to read the Qur'an and to interpret Islamic texts on a range of moral issues. These schools still exist. Thus while formal education in southwestern Nigeria (and in southern Nigeria more generally) derives mainly from the West, in Northern Nigeria text-based education has historically centered on the Qur'an, the Hadith, and other Islamic books, mainly from the Middle East.

These educational and religious affiliations have, to a great extent, affected general attitudes toward the West and toward Western ideas and things. A range of Western educational, technological, and biomedical practices, including polio vaccination, has been widely accepted in southern Nigeria, where people look to the West as a source of progress for themselves and their communities.[14] In Northern Nigeria, however, people have often been suspicious of things introduced from the West, from bicycles to Western education to contraceptives (Renne 1996). While many Northern Nigerian children now attend primary and secondary schools as well as colleges and universities which offer Western education, this attendance grew slowly, after initial suspicions were quelled. Nonetheless, the many children who attend schools offering Western education also go to schools providing Islamic education. It should not be surprising, then, that suspicions about polio vaccines were voiced by Islamiyya teachers, whose schools are instrumental to the continuation of a particular social order in Northern Nigerian communities in which Islamic faith and practice are paramount (M. Last 2008).

The distrust felt by these men (and others) was voiced in terms of contaminated oral polio vaccine. A wide range of Northern Nigerian Muslims, from university professors to politicians, expressed fears of such contamination, suggesting some of the ways that religion may become openly intertwined with politics (Obadare 2005). Apprehension about Western biomedicine was also reinforced by the 1996 Trovan drug trial in Kano, discussed in chapter 7. However, this distrust of the oral polio vaccine was not entirely unfounded, considering the subsequent 2005 outbreak of circulating vaccine-derived poliovirus (CDC 2007a, 2007b, 2009a; WHO 2007d). Although the outbreak was not caused by contaminated oral polio vaccine, it resulted from the reversion of type 2 Sabin vaccine into virulent strains of poliovirus.

Polio, Paralysis, and Disability

While the political aspects of public health campaigns should not be ignored, the consequences of contracting a particular disease and how this situation is interpreted also need to be considered within a particular cultural context. The primary visibly distinguishing symptom of poliomyelitis in children is acute flaccid paralysis. However, very few children five years old or younger experience paralysis. Rather, most children in Northern Nigeria experience polio as a fever or cold. Yet the question of why one child who is infected with the poliovirus becomes paralyzed when others do not may be explained in different ways, reflecting more general cultural views about illness and disease causation.

In Northern Nigeria, paralysis has historically been associated with the presence of spirits (Wall 1988). While the specific identity of these spirits has changed over time, their presence and the paralysis associated with them is viewed as deriving from God (M. Last 1967), as are the medicines and treatments that will bring about cure. This perception of illness and medicine affects the treatment of those who are paralyzed and whether paralysis is perceived as a stigma, as something destined by God, or as something else. It also affects people's ideas about the prevention of diseases such as polio, about polio immunization, about the disabled and how they should be treated, and about what constitutes a disability (Geurts 2002; Holzer, Vreede, and Weigt 1999; Ingstad and Whyte 1995). For how disability is addressed in any society reflects these larger socioeconomic and cultural frames. In the West, individuals disabled by disease or accident are seen as the responsibility of the secular state as well as of their families. In Hausa society, until recently, the disabled received minimal or no assistance from the state. Rather, they were supported through the religious obligation of alms-giving and a well-organized social system of begging.[15]

In the past, a lame male child (*gurgu*) had a particular social role. Since such boys were rarely able to work as farmers or traders, their families expected that they would beg for a living.[16] Several older Hausa men who had worked as beggars in various Nigerian cities for most of their lives told me that they would have preferred other occupations, but that begging was the only form of work available to them. Yet if paralysis and subsequent lameness are explained as coming from God, this work makes sense in the larger framework of Hausa Muslim obligations and alms-giving.

While such children might receive an Islamic education, they were rarely able to attend schools providing Western education. In the past, a parent who wanted to send a child to such a school would be opposed by family members who viewed such an expenditure as a costly extravagance when a disabled child could be earning his keep by begging. However, some children paralyzed as a result of polio have experienced their condition and its association with begging as stigmatizing, in the sense described by Goffman (1973). Such a stigma—associated with socially denigrated categories of persons whose identities contrast with social ideals—may be overcome in various ways, such as by hiding a disability. While such strategies are not available to those with severe paralysis, some are attempting to diminish the stigma of the association of lameness with begging by pursuing higher education. Their reassessment of a certain social trajectory is paralleled by their putting pressure on government agencies to provide services, with some measure of success, and their support for efforts to prevent polio.

Thus in Northern Nigeria stigma is associated with begging, not with being disabled per se, so that polio and its aftermath are not pressing concerns, especially when social and political organizations offer occupational alternatives. This is not to romanticize or trivialize the difficulties of the lame in Hausa society, but rather to show how long-standing ideas about paralysis and its socioeconomic consequences intersect with parents' assessments of the relative risks of polio and the oral polio vaccine.

The Ethics of Polio Eradication in Northern Nigeria

If parents' distrust of the polio vaccine and of the motives of those promoting the Polio Eradication Initiative stemmed in part from the Initiative's exclusive focus on polio, this single-mindedness was not the original intention of the World Health Assembly (WHA 1988a). For when the World Health Assembly resolved in 1988 to implement an initiative to eradicate poliomyelitis globally, it was noted "that efforts to eradicate poliomyelitis [will] serve to strengthen other immunization and health services, especially those for women and children" (WHA 1988b). Yet in Northern Nigeria, rather than strengthening "other immunization and health services, especially those for women and children," as the World Health Assembly document prescribed, the Polio Eradication Initiative appears to have "contribut[ed] to the continuing dysfunction of the primary health care system" (FBA Health Systems Analysts 2005, v), at least initially, by concentrating community health personnel's time and resources on polio vaccination during National Immunization Days.[17] On the one hand, many Northern Nigerians questioned the ethics of a health campaign which failed to "help . . . people who are sick [at the hospital]" and "just focus[ed] on polio" (interview, Zaria, 31 August 2005), seeing it as a top-down government decision to promote a public health initiative that had relatively little relevance to their children's health. While people's protests against the Polio Eradication Initiative were widely decried as ignorant and unethical by international public health officials and by the Western press, Northern Nigerians' criticisms of the Initiative as an inappropriate health intervention, whether directly stated as a waste of health care funds for a minor health problem or couched in terms of rumors about infertility and HIV-AIDS, voiced legitimate concerns.

On the other hand, national and international public health officials, anxious to eradicate polio and the unnecessary suffering it caused paralyzed victims, saw this focus as the only means of accomplishing this end. From their perspective, public health personnel questioned the ethics of parents in Northern Nigeria, where wild poliovirus is endemic, who refused to immunize their children against polio and who thereby undermined efforts to raise community immunity to a high level, referred to as "herd immunity," when enough children have been immunized that disease transmission is slowed or stopped (Parry et al. 2004, 139). Their refusal not only provided a viral reservoir from which the wild poliovirus could be spread to other countries, both within and outside of Africa (CDC 2006b), but also contributed to low immunization levels that fostered the spread of circulating vaccine-derived polioviruses (CDC 2007a, 2007b). For Ministry of Health officials, and major donors, such as Rotary International, their position was the ethical one.

Yet one might ask, if the World Health Assembly included the strengthening of primary health care along with polio eradication in its 1988 resolution and if prominent public health professionals, seeing the results of earlier polio eradication efforts in Latin America, were warning about the consequences of eradication efforts in countries with weak health infrastructures (e.g., Taylor, Cutts, and Taylor 1997), why were these concerns not taken into account in the Nigerian Polio Eradication Initiative? Henderson (1998) refers to the "siren song of eradication," arguing that donors and public health personnel alike are seduced by the challenge of a campaign to eradicate a particular disease and forget, as they did in the case of polio eradication, about the importance of basic primary health care for their campaign's success. Furthermore, rather than tailoring interventions to specific situations, as in countries with weak health infrastructures and sub-populations with particular experiences of colonialism and postcolonial rule, officials confronting the demanding logistics of conducting an eradication campaign favored the development of a uniform protocol which could be used universally. In such public health campaigns, there is a tendency to focus on the disease—which is viewed as acultural—rather than on the cultural, social, and historical particularities of the different societies concerned (Kunitz 2006).

However, there are also economic and political reasons for this trend toward focusing on a specific disease or health problem, having to do with shifts in public health policies and in the provision of health care that support this approach.

In recent years, donors and international agencies have come to prefer health interventions with a specific goal and time frame, which they view as "economical as well as humane" (Kunitz 1987, 396). Hardon and Blume (2005, 348) have noted a general ideological shift from the broad-based health projects of the 1980s that were implemented through primary health care programs—such as the Expanded Programme on Immunisation—to an emphasis on disease eradication and technological innovation, represented by the Polio Eradication Initiative in the 1990s. This shift also reflects economic considerations, since time-bound interventions such as the polio eradication campaign are seen as more cost-effective than open-ended ones (S. Barrett 2004), and hence are more attractive to donors (Kunitz 1987). For organizations such as Rotary International, which had raised nearly US$644 million for polio eradication worldwide as of 2007 (WHO 2007a) and was awarded a matching grant of US$100 million by the Gates Foundation in the same year (Dugger 2007), such projects generate activism among members and provide a focus for fundraising. Indeed, broad-based programs, such as the Expanded Programme on Immunisation, that are carried out through a system of primary health care hospitals and clinics have difficulty maintaining long-term financial sustainability.

Yet this strategy of fundraising has ethical and logistical dimensions, as Taylor, Cutts, and Taylor (1997, 922) have noted with respect to the Polio Eradication Initiative:

> A basic policy question is, How will global goals and local priorities be balanced, and what are the ethical implications of current choices? The specific underlying questions are as follows: Should poor countries, with many health problems that could be controlled, divert their limited resources for a global goal that has low priority for their own children? When wild virus remains only in a few sites, will rich countries, and the global organizations they influence, promote eradication as a single-focus activity? Should poor countries expect donors to improve upon past experience and use the opportunity and financial benefits from polio eradication to build sustainable health systems for the world's neediest children?

By concentrating on polio eradication without providing affordable primary health care, the national government and international funding agencies essentially placed the responsibility of health care on individuals and their families. Northern Nigerians who protested against the Polio Eradication Initiative insisted that if they were to accept the polio vaccination for their children, then the government had to provide primary health care and other basic services. With the implementation of Immunization Plus Days in 2006, their demands were recognized and partially met. Yet their protests might have been foreseen if Polio Eradication Initiative officials had been willing to test their immunization protocol in areas such as Northern Nigeria, where resistance to Western products and other Western-based health initiatives was well known, before implementing a full-fledged campaign (Lubeck 1985; Miller, Barrett, and Henderson 2006, 1174; Renne 1996; see also Feldman-Savelsberg, Ndonko, and Schmidt-Ehry 2000).

Under pressure to raise funds from donors for an eradication program, Polio Eradication Initiative officials overlooked the long-term consequences of a weak health infrastructure, including the difficulties of establishing a well-organized surveillance system and an active program of laboratory research (Henderson 1999), and may thereby have hampered the Initiative's progress in Northern Nigeria.

*   *   *

The rumors which circulated in Northern Nigeria concerning the polio vaccine, that it was contaminated by infertility drugs or by HIV-AIDS, suggest other rumors, in other times and places, associated with public fears about disruptive social and economic changes and with an influx of foreign things and people (M. Last 2008). Philip Kuhn, for example, describes the widespread rumors of disappearing queues and stolen souls in eighteenth-century China, during the late imperial period, when rumor provided a principal form of expression for ordinary people who lacked political power (Kuhn 1990, 230). In Northern Nigeria, rumors about polio vaccine and other Western products, such as Panadol (a brand of paracetamol, or acetaminophen) and Maggi brand bouillon cubes (Renne 1996), also reflect concerns about maintaining the integrity of the Muslim community—the *dar al-Islam,* the "house of Islam" (M. Last 2008, 46)—which consists of a complex of cultural and social practices, including knowledge of the Qur'an, gender mores, and alms-giving, as well as Hausa medicine and language. For many, Islam provides a guide to ethical conduct and an antidote to fears about the hegemony of Western ideas, practices, and things. Furthermore, the genuine concerns of some parents that the polio vaccine could be harmful to their children's fertility also bespeaks greater fears about national political marginalization, about a continuing decline in primary health care, and about a general insecurity in Nigeria and in the world.

This book considers this social dynamic in one society in West Africa, although people's fears for the future may be seen in many other societies as well. Northern Nigeria's particular historical experiences—as a center of trade and Islamic learning, as a strong opponent of British and Christian colonial conquest in the early twentieth century, and as the home of a large and diverse population, which is primarily united by Islam—have contributed to how its people perceive their position vis à vis the Nigerian state and the West. Their experiences of illness and epidemics are also distinctive: malaria, measles, and cerebrospinal meningitis are the diseases that preoccupy them. The frightening polio epidemics experienced in the U.S. during the first half of the twentieth century did not occur in Northern Nigeria. Indeed, during the 1950s, when polio vaccine trials were being conducted in the U.S. (Francis et al. 1957; Oshinsky 2005), British colonial officials in Nigeria, while supporting polio vaccination for expatriates, viewed Nigerians as having "natural immunity" and thus not requiring vaccination (Familusi and Adesina 1977). It was not until almost fifty years later that polio vaccination of Nigerians was viewed as a critical concern. Northern Nigerians' historical experiences—of polio; of emirate, colonial, and federal rule; and of Islamic religious practice—within the particular sociocultural and political context during which the Polio Eradication Initiative was implemented have contributed to their distinctive response to this campaign.

*　　*　　*

This book is based on research conducted primarily in Northern Nigeria, in the town of Zaria in northern Kaduna State. In September 1994, I came to Zaria as a Fulbright Fellow to teach at Ahmadu Bello University. In October 1994, I took up residence in a family home in the section of Zaria known as Zaria City or Birnin Zazzau, where I first met my neighbor, the father of the young boy described at the beginning of this chapter, and where I have resided for at least two weeks every year over the past fifteen years. This long-term field work was crucial for this research project, as without it I would have been unable to discuss issues surrounding the controversial Polio Eradication Initiative with a range of individuals. Beginning in 2005, I have spoken with parents who did or did not have their children vaccinated for polio, with individuals who had had polio or with their parents, with immunization workers, with local government health officials, and with primary and secondary school teachers and Islamic scholars. Nor would I have been able to ask whether marks on houses indicating that they had been visited by health care workers on National Immunization Days actually meant that polio vaccines had been given, and to be told the truth. My connections with Ahmadu Bello University also facilitated interviews with public health professors, pediatricians, and pharmacologists. It was through these connections that I spoke with a professor emeritus who specialized in polio research at the University of Ibadan; with the acting director of the Office of Special Education, Ministry of Education, Kaduna State; with three members of the WHO Polio Eradication Initiative team, and with the head of the Kaduna State National Programme on Immunization, all headquartered in Kaduna. In addition, I have read articles on the polio campaign published in two Northern Nigerian newspapers, *The Weekly Trust* and *The Daily Trust,* from May 2003 to June 2009, which are held at Arewa House (a Northern Nigerian research center in Kaduna) and are available online, and have examined newspaper clippings and unpublished materials on earlier immunization efforts in Nigeria that are held in the library of the Department of Community Medicine, Ahmadu Bello University, in the Nigerian National Archives—Kaduna, and in the Ahmadu Bello University Kashim Ibrahim Library. These interviews and written texts were complemented by everyday observations of sayings and slogans painted on the backs of buses and on city walls, of radio spots, of fashions in dress,[18] and of popular songs. Taken together, these sources document the particular course the Polio Eradication Initiative has taken in Northern Nigeria.

2.   Smallpox and Polio Histories

When we held the *bori* dance here at New Giwa, Inna, the Fulani woman came, she was coaxed and persuaded to come. Two *bori* dancers . . . went to her tree in the middle of the night and fetched her. . . . Inna is lame, so they went to fetch her with something to carry her back in.

—Smith, *Baba of Karo*

We would do these vaccinations when there was an outbreak of smallpox. Some people refused it, especially the *malamai* [Islamic teachers], who said that there must be a motive behind it. The *mai anguwai* [neighborhood leaders] would get people together to support immunization.

—Alhaji Yusufu Abdullahi, Kaduna

In Nigeria, there have been two major disease eradication campaigns—one aimed at smallpox, which was begun in 1967 and concluded in 1970 (Fenner et al. 1988), and more recently one aimed at polio, which was begun in 1996 and is ongoing. How Western medicine was received, whether presented as prevention or treatment, depended on whether these campaigns coincided with or countered prevailing explanatory and classificatory schemes of the disease in question, what Rosenberg (1992) refers to as "disease frames." A comparison of the different cultural, social, and epidemiological histories of smallpox and polio as well as efforts to contain them underscores the ways that the conceptual framing of these diseases and their particular etiologies contributed to or hindered these initiatives. That smallpox was widely known among Northern Nigerians is suggested by the number of names given to it—*agana* (smallpox), *'yan rani* (child of the dry season), and *cin zanzana* (eating pockmarks, which are also referred to as *ado*, decoration). That it was considered to be a dangerous disease is suggested by the name *cin zanzana*, as the Hausa verb *ci* is widely used in other semantic constructions that involve appropriation and conquest (Gouffé 1966, 94–95). A range of therapies were associated with smallpox, including spirit possession, prayers and amulets, herbal medications, and inoculation, which indicate its significance in Hausa society in the past. This past framing of the disease of *agana* by Northern Nigerians parallels and even coincides with British colonial and international health workers' conceptions of the disease called smallpox. While their explanations of the etiology of this disease differed, their assessment of its deadly contagiousness and the use, by some, of vaccination and inoculation were similar. Resistance to smallpox vaccination did not derive from different understandings of the disease but reflected other, more political, concerns—e.g., fears of European rulers' motives, challenges to Western assertions of medical superiority, and preferences for local institutions and practices. Yet many agreed with British colonial officials' and, later, international health workers' assessment of this disease and supported the campaign for its eradication.

By contrast, the term Shan Inna (or "polio," the term used by younger people) refers generally to paralysis, which may be attributed to a number of diseases, including polio but also Guillain-Barré syndrome. Historically, Shan Inna was addressed through spiritual as well as medicinal means. No preventative measures such as inoculation were taken. This lack of specificity of disease naming, prevention, and treatment coincided with colonial officials' lack of concern with poliomyelitis as a public health problem for Nigerians, although in the 1950s they hastened to provide the recently available Salk vaccine to colonial expatriate staff and their families. It was not until the 1980s, with the inclusion of polio vaccine in the Expanded Programme on Immunisation, and the 1990s, with the commencement of the Polio Eradication Initiative, that polio was represented as a dangerous childhood disease in Nigeria. That many Northern Nigerian parents did not redefine polio in this way, continuing to view it as a relatively minor affliction, underscores the disjuncture of views between many Northern Nigerians and Western and Western-trained public health officials. An examination of Hausa medicine, its practice as well as its underlying logic, helps to explain the similarities, differences, and transformations in disease frames and their consequences for smallpox and polio eradication efforts.

Hausa Medical Practice

In Northern Nigeria, treatments for a range of diseases have been available to Hausa healing specialists, who rely on a vast pharmacopoeia of herbal medicines (Dalziel 1916; Etkin 1981; Jinju 1990; Oliver-Bever 1986; Wall 1988), as well as to Muslim teachers (*malamai*), who utilize their particular knowledge of prayer and associated techniques (Wall 1988). They use a variety of herbal medicines, spiritual rituals, written and spoken suras from the Qur'an, and, more recently, Western pharmaceuticals, as well as surgical techniques, to bring about cure (Etkin 1992; Etkin, Ross, and Muazzamu 1990; Wall 1988). In some instances, they will use preventive techniques, such as variolation for smallpox (Herbert 1975) or the ingestion of sour things to reduce the impact of a condition referred to as "sweet" during pregnancy (Trevitt 1973). However, paralysis, which did not readily respond to treatment, was attributed to spiritual beings, known as *bori* spirits. By performing rituals to appease Shan Inna, seen as the spirit responsible for paralytic polio, the afflicted and their families sought to bring about cure. Such an approach to illness makes sense in Hausa society, where medical explanations are holistic and include spiritual as well as physical sources of illness. Indeed, although the practice of *bori* spirit possession has declined, particularly in urban areas in Northern Nigeria where stricter forms of Islam, which forbid traditional religious practices, have increasing numbers of followers, illness may be attributed to other spirits (often called *aljanu*, jinn or genie) that are mentioned in the Qur'an (see Soares 2005), as evidenced by the ritual exorcism (*rukiyya*) of such spirits (O'Brien 2001).

Nonetheless, a certain amount of pragmatism was involved when cure was not obtained through local methods. During the colonial period, the sick might be taken to a local clinic or hospital where Western medical treatment was available. Indeed, some traditional Hausa healers (but not all) have incorporated Western pharmaceuticals—tablets, antibiotic ointments, and sometimes injectibles—into their healing practices, interpreting their curative properties according to their own medical rubric (Etkin, Ross, and Muazzamu 1990). Thus, when the situation warrants, both "modern" Western and "traditional" Hausa medications may be seen as appropriate. The reception of Western medicine also depended on circumstances. During epidemics, people were more amenable to trying Western care, particularly when local medicines and treatments were ineffective.

The intersection of Hausa and Western medicine mainly began in the colonial period, although European travelers in the nineteenth century frequently mention giving medicines upon request and as gifts.[1] However, after the defeat of the army of the Sultan of Sokoto in 1903, broad sections of the population were exposed to Western medicines and medical practices, as colonial officials attempted to control the transmission of infectious diseases. This exchange of ideas and *materia medica* has continued through to the present, when people have recourse to a range of Western and traditional Hausa medicines in their quest for cure (Janzen 1978).

Knowledge of Smallpox and Its Treatment

During the precolonial and early colonial period (and probably earlier), smallpox (*agana* or *cin zanzana*) and cerebrospinal meningitis were responsible for major epidemics in Northern Nigeria (Herbert 1975; Horn 1951; Wall 1988). Heinrich Barth, for example, who traveled extensively in West Africa during the 1850s, mentions smallpox "as a very fatal disease in Central Africa" (1857, 1:338). Considered to be a "hot" disease, it was treated with "cooling medicines" that would take away the heat of the smallpox pustules, such as poultices made from honey (Clapperton 1829, 2:76; Wall 1988, 298) and from the plant *babba juji* (*Boerhaavia diffusa*)[2] (Ayensu 1978, 201; Dalziel 1916, 11), which would assuage itching. One older man in Zaria described his sister's treatment for smallpox (*agana*), probably in the 1930s:

> I had *agana* and my sister had *agana* . . . but my own was not much. My sister's was much and she has the marks on her face—the smallpox spoiled her face. At that time, they used one leaf called *saniya kasa* and *kashin* [dung] from camels; they mixed it together and they would bathe you in this mixture. And sometimes they would heat sand and ask a person to lie down on it because if the smallpox is too much, the pustules will stick to the [sleeping] mat. (Interview, Yakasai, 3 August 2006)

Smallpox was also associated with *bori* spirits, although how these particular spirits were represented and treated in Northern Nigeria is not well documented.[3] *Bori* dances were performed for smallpox victims, who were known as Yayan zanzanna, "children of smallpox" (Onwuejeogwu 1969, 288; Treamearne 1914).

However, some groups in Northern Nigeria also used preventive practices to reduce the risk of full-blown cases of smallpox. Prophylactic inoculation (variolation) for smallpox was recorded in Northern Nigeria during the nineteenth century by Barth (1857), Clapperton (1829), and Denham and Clapperton (1826).[4] Individuals inoculated with smallpox experienced smallpox symptoms, but usually had milder cases of the disease and died less frequently. While powdered smallpox scabs (inhaled or placed in cuts on the body) have been used elsewhere, in Northern Nigeria fluid from smallpox vesicles was placed on cuts on the forearms (Foy 1915; Meek 1931; Pifer and Adeoye 1968).[5] Baba of Karo described how such inoculation was done in the area around Kano during the late nineteenth century:

> They used to scratch your arm until the blood came, then they got the fluid from someone who had the smallpox and rubbed it in. It all swelled up and you covered it until it healed. Some children used to die; your way of doing it is better. (Smith 1954, 46)

As Baba noted, although fluid was taken from those suffering mild cases of smallpox, the strength of the virus varied and the resulting case of smallpox could sometimes cause serious illness or death. The use of cowpox lymph, first tested by Edward Jenner in 1796, was the better way of doing it to which Baba refers.

Colonial Concerns and Smallpox Immunization Campaigns (1903–1960)

With the commencement of British colonial rule in Northern Nigeria in 1903, government officials had to address major and recurrent epidemics of smallpox on a shoestring budget.[6] British colonial officials introduced the use of dried cowpox lymph in 1903 in Northern Nigeria, although the viability of the lymph was so poor that vaccination offered little protection against smallpox. While the introduction of imported lanolinated calf lymph in 1921 improved vaccination success rates somewhat, the practice was resisted in both southern and Northern Nigeria. Resistance in southwestern Nigeria reflected traditional religious beliefs associated with Shopona, the smallpox deity, although resistance was eventually reduced by police orders.[7] By 1921, 297,823 individuals were reported to have been vaccinated for smallpox in southern Nigeria.[8] Resistance in the North was due mainly to fear of Europeans and their medicine and possibly to some groups' preference for local methods of inoculation.[9] This resistance, along with the vast size of the Northern Province and the inadequate health resources of the colonial medical service, resulted in considerably fewer smallpox vaccinations being carried out there. In 1921, for example, only 15,731 vaccinations were recorded, only 5.3 percent of the number vaccinated in the south in the same year.

Despite local inoculation for smallpox and continued efforts at smallpox vaccination by the colonial medical service, smallpox epidemics continued in Northern Nigeria during the first half of the twentieth century.[10] The colonial administration continued to try various techniques to improve immunization levels, including the introduction of a vaccination ordinance in 1917.[11] In 1945, the ordinance was amended to include a schedule for compulsory vaccination of adults and children, to be organized by local political authorities (Jakeway 1945). These Native Authority officials were also responsible for determining penalties for noncooperation, although specific fines for noncompliance were subsequently introduced (Compulsory Vaccination in Northern Provinces, Nigerian National Archives).

While colonial government officials could draft ordinances to compel traditional rulers to enforce vaccination in their areas of jurisdiction, one gets a better sense of how the postwar vaccination campaigns were carried out in Northern Nigeria by examining the archival reports of expatriate medical doctors and Nigerian vaccination team members (dressers, sanitary inspectors). In one case in 1949, in the area of Takum in the part of the Northern Province now known as Taraba State,

> some of the villages would not respond favourably to vaccination. At the mere notice or sight of our arrival most of the village heads and their people would run away and hid themselves on farms and bushes in the hilly countryside. . . . .In some cases we had to threaten carrying away their village and hamlet heads to Wukari where coaxing and explanations failed but in some others like Kpambo and Lissan, no amount of tact would induce most of them to present themselves for vaccination. . . . .A list of the names of the Village heads and Sub-heads of Kpambo and Lissan has been submitted to the Sarkin Takum for prosecution at his demand after having heard our verbal report. (Report by a government sanitary inspector, Wukari, 11 November 1949, in Vaccination Campaign Reports, Nigerian National Archives)

In another case, in the Sokoto Emirate in the northwestern part of the Northern Province, a campaign was carried out from June to October 1951, with the approval of the local Native Authority ruler, the Sultan of Sokoto:

> Dressers in charge of teams were instructed to render weekly progress reports, and the work of the teams was closely supervised. The problem of checking results proved to be very difficult, because the people, afraid of being revaccinated, failed to come up for inspection. In spite of this, several controls were made during the vaccination period. The teams, besides being equipped with routine vaccination outfits were supplied with dressings, simple drugs etc, because the people in isolated villages begged for attention to their ulcers, septic eyes, injuries etc, etc. In general the villagers were very reluctant to attend for vaccination, and in many places the influence of the Sultan's representative was not sufficiently strong to persuade the people that vaccination is for their benefit.

This officer also made a point of noting the importance of Nigerian team members, whose good work facilitated vaccination:

Here the writer wishes to commend the Dressers for their work. Many of them proved to be full of initiative and energy in their work. In many instances they stimulated the District Head or NA representatives for a more active attitude towards the campaign. They trekked hundreds of miles and visited hundreds of villages; at the same time, they inspected houses and carried out health propaganda. For instance, one of the dressers trying hard to secure the attendance of the people says in his report, "I have been preaching the Gospel of vaccination to the people, and the same time telling them the evil of smallpox." (V. Romanowski, medical officer, 16 November 1951, in Vaccination Campaign Reports, Nigerian National Archives)

While views of smallpox vaccination may be indirectly gleaned from these colonial government reports, it is difficult to know how to assess the dresser's mention of "preaching," what house inspection consisted of, or how effective these vaccination efforts were.

With increasing numbers of vaccinations being carried out, there was also a large increase in the number of cases of smallpox, as judged by the evidence of pockmark scars. In 1949, 21,559 cases were reported, compared to 5,746 cases reported in 1948. However, it was not entirely clear how this difference should be interpreted. In 1952 the acting director of medical services for the Northern Region argued,

Too much reliance must not be placed on figures for the incidence of the disease or the number of vaccinations performed which are shown in the Annual Reports of the Department. In fact the only inference I am prepared to draw is that smallpox is still endemic in the North. I am not prepared to admit at this stage that this disease is on the increase. It is significant to note that the number of reported cases has been rising annually since 1948. This corresponds to the series of large scale meningitis epidemics[12] to which so much publicity was given, during which so much propaganda was done and which were tackled so successfully by the Field Units, that Village and District Heads have realized the importance of notification of infectious diseases and are now conscientiously reporting cases as soon as they occur. This, in my opinion, is the main reason for the continuing rise in reported cases. (J. P. Sexton, Kaduna, in Vaccination Campaign Reports, Nigerian National Archives)

Nonetheless, despite increased vaccination numbers, cases of smallpox may indeed have increased during the late 1940s and 1950s, because of the quality of the lymph used (Henry 1955). After 1921, lanolinated calf lymph was imported from the British Lister Institute which, due to shipment and climatic factors, was of variable potency. Consequently, attempts were then made to manufacture lanolinated sheep lymph in Nigeria, and in 1941, the colonial Laboratory Service in Yaba, Lagos, supplied smallpox vaccine for the entire country (Horn 1952). This vaccine, however, was sensitive to heat, and under unrefrigerated conditions could lose its potency. A pockmark survey carried out during the Smallpox Eradication Program led researchers to estimate that 100,000 or more cases had occurred in Nigeria annually during the early 1960s (Fenner et al 1988, 882), seeming to indicate a large increase in cases. Population growth may also have increased the incidence of both smallpox and poliomyelitis during this period.

Poliomyelitis, Polio, Shan Inna

Like smallpox, during the precolonial and early colonial periods paralytic poliomyelitis was associated with a particular *bori* spirit, the lame Fulani woman Shan Inna mentioned by Baba of Karo. She was said to drink (*sha*) the blood of her victims' atrophied limbs. Treatment consisted of offerings to this spirit as well as prayers and various sorts of herbal infusions and poultices. Since the acute flaccid paralysis linked with polio is also a symptom of other neuropathological conditions (Hull 2004, 698; Marx, Glass, and Sutter 2000), paralysis was sometimes temporary. Hence treatment through *bori* possession could be seen as therapeutic, lending support to *bori* spirit healers' claims of cure.[13]

One elderly man presently living in Zaria who had had polio as a child in Zamfara State described treatment by a *bori* specialist after herbal treatments by traditional healers had failed, probably in the early 1920s:

> There was a time, one *bori* woman said she could give me medicine that will cure me. My father asked her to come and gave her a room to stay in the house. My father said he would do everything she wanted. I was sleeping in the room my father gave to her and she was giving me medicine. She said I will definitely walk but at the time I stood up, nobody should say anything.
>
> One time when we were playing with some children, around 9 PM in the night. . . . When we were playing with these children, I forgot that I was disabled, then I stood up. Then my mother started shouting, "He's standing up! He's standing up!" From that time, I just fell down. Since that time I never stood up again.
>
> At that time my father came, he wanted to beat my mother. There was one imam from our mosque who came to our house that time, he was the one who said that my father should not beat my mother. But the *bori* woman said to my mother, "You spoiled my medicine!" She went out and disappeared. Nobody knew where she went. (Interview, Zaria, 10 August 2005)

This case, in which a woman whose authority rested on her association with *bori* spirits also prepared medicines for her patient, underscores both the spiritual and physiological dimensions by which the boy's condition was understood. Another interesting aspect of this story is his father's acceptance of *bori* healing as well as the advice of the imam, suggesting that the line between reliance on traditional spiritual cures and Islam was not so severely drawn as it is in Zaria presently. Thus, while polio continues to be known as Shan Inna, many younger people in Zaria today do not know that the name refers to a *bori* spirit, in part because *bori* worship has been discouraged by Muslim leaders as an un-Islamic practice. After the British colonial government was established in 1903, British officials also disapproved of *bori* spiritual practices,[14] which nonetheless have continued, particularly in rural areas of Northern Nigeria (Yahya 2007).

Treatment of Polio during the Colonial Period

In contrast to smallpox, with which colonial officials were concerned from early on, polio was not considered an urgent health problem, to judge by archival records. Indeed, it was only in the late 1950s and after Independence, during the early 1960s, that researchers began to study the prevalence of polio-myelitis among Nigerians (Collis et al. 1961).[15]

However, an increase in the incidence of polio among expatriates during the 1950s led to a growing concern with polio vaccination, which the recent introduction of the Salk polio vaccine made possible. This increase was a consequence of the particular epidemiology of the poliovirus, which is spread through fecal-oral transmission. In countries without sewage systems or easy access to clean water, individuals are often exposed to the virus as infants, after the initial short-term immunity derived from their mothers wears off. But those who have grown up in hygienic environments where exposure to poliovirus is unlikely, such as Great Britain during the early twentieth century, may contract life-threatening cases of paralytic polio as adolescents and adults (Paul 1971, 365). In Nigeria, "six adult Europeans" contracted polio in Lagos during the first six months of 1956, and at least two expatriates died from polio, one in 1947 and another in 1958 (Poliomy-elitis, Nigerian National Archives; Gardner-Brown, 26 June 1956, in Salk Anti-poliomyelitis Vaccine, Nigerian National Archives).

Colonial Office personnel in London were especially concerned by the prospect of notifying new unvaccinated recruits about the possibility of contracting polio "at a time when recruitment to Nigeria is already so difficult" (A. R. Thomas to A. Gardner-Brown, 1956, in Salk Anti-poliomyelitis Vaccine, Nigerian National Archives).[16] Fearing that nondisclosure of the polio danger would make matters worse, and because so little was known about polio in Nigeria, by 1957 they had instituted a scheme for vaccinating the following categories of people:[17]

1) Expatriate children or Nigerian children born outside West Africa, as well as expatriate nursing sisters and laboratory superintendents . . . ,
2) Expatriate children in Nigeria from 1 year up, who have not been previously vaccinated,
3) Pregnant expatriate women, and
4) Other expatriates. (Director of medical services, Northern Region, 29 July 1957, in Salk Anti-poliomyelitis Vaccine, Nigerian National Archives)

The danger of expatriates' acquiring polio persuaded officials at the Colonial Office to obtain more information about poliomyelitis in Nigeria. Dr. J. C. R. Bucanan promised, "On the medical side I will try and get some chapter and verse on incidence rates and other technical points from one or two selected territories. We really know very little about the endemic position [of polio] in Africa and elsewhere" (11 July 1956, in Salk Anti-poliomyelitis Vaccine, Nigerian National Archives). Consequently, two studies were carried out in 1955 and 1956, one in Lagos by the chief medical adviser, who examined blood serum from twenty-six children for polio antibodies, and another in the village of Kadandani (south of Katsina), this one a study of 348 individuals by Dr. J. S. Gear in cooperation with the World Health Organization. In both studies, the incidence of polio antibodies was found to be high in all subjects except newborns, indicating that they had been exposed to the poliomyelitis virus.[18]

These small studies confirmed the belief of colonial officials that Nigerians had "natural immunity" and hence did not need protection through vaccination. Thus in 1955 the director of medical services, Northern Region, wrote,

> In the last Annual Report published, i.e., for 1953–4, two cases only [of poliomyelitis] were reported in the Northern Region. The figures for 1954–55, among others, are still in process of collation, and are not yet available. This year (1955–56) only one case has so far been recorded. In view of these facts . . . it is considered unwise at this stage to carry a stock of prophylactic vaccine against poliomyelitis. (23 May 1955, Kaduna, in Poliomyelitis, Nigerian National Archives)

However, with several cases of polio reported for the period from 1947 to 1959 in Northern Nigeria (in Katsina, Zaria, Dutsen Wai, Garkida, Kafanchan, Ilorin, Jos, Yola, Kano, and Maiduguri), colonial medical personnel began to revise this assessment. In May 1959, the permanent secretary for the Ministry of Health wrote to senior medical officers in the North,

> From the casual observation of paralised men and children in Kaduna, Kano & Ilorin, I have the impression that paralitic Poliomyelitic [sic] amongst young Africans is a great deal more common [than] notifications suggest: in fact I have the impression that it is a common disease, rarely notified.
>   It is of great importance for the framing of future policy for preventative medicine to get some idea of the true picture of this disease in Northern Nigeria. I should therefore be glad if the greatest care could be taken in future of the prompt and accurate notification of poliomyelitis. (30 May 1959, in Poliomyelitis Inoculation, Nigerian National Archives)

This reassessment of the prevalence of poliomyelitis among Nigerian children was reinforced by a hospital-based study of admissions to the newly opened Children's Neurology Clinic at University College Hospital–Ibadan (Collis et al. 1961). During the period from 1958 to 1960, 350 cases of poliomyelitis (mainly in children from the Ibadan areas, but also in those from other Nigerian towns) were diagnosed, with the majority of cases between 1 and 3 years of age and with 95 out of 314 suffering paralysis of one or both legs (Collis et al. 1961, 219).[19] In a report presented at the conference on childhood infectious diseases held in Lagos in January 1961, Collis observed that "he had been told that poliomyelitis was no problem at the University College Hospital, Ibadan, among the African population but in the Clinic we found at once that this was quite incorrect and that by far the largest group of neurological conditions in childhood is caused by the poliomyelitis viruses." In fact, "there are a minimum of 100,000 cripples of all ages from poliomyelitis in Nigeria" (Collis et al. 1961, 217, 222). Familusi and Adesina, in their study of 2,063 case records of children diagnosed with poliomyelitis at University College Hospital–Ibadan from January 1964 to December 1973, found that poliomyelitis was prevalent in the Ibadan area throughout the year, without relation to season or temperature. They attributed this prevalence to increasing population and urban crowding, along with an incomplete course or total lack of polio immunization. While cases declined from September 1964 to August 1965, probably because of a mass campaign against polio carried out by the World Health Organization in Ibadan in August and September 1964 using oral polio vaccine, after this brief immunization effort the number of cases presenting to University College Hospital continued to increase (Familusi and Adesina 1977, 121).

With such large numbers of children affected by poliomyelitis, the possibility of immunization was raised. Since polio vaccines were relatively new at this time, there were questions not only about whether to vaccinate Nigerian children from six months to five years of age, but also about the type of vaccine to use. Both Collis et al. (1961) and Stones (1961) recommended vaccination of Nigerian children using the oral attenuated Sabin vaccine:

> If there is anywhere in the world where the live virus could be used with success it should be in Nigeria. The introduction of an avirulent strain here could not conceivably make the situation worse even if it regained some virulence by passage. Clearly this is a matter for careful approach and control but the issue should be squarely and immediately faced. (Collis et al. 1961, 222)

Alternatively, Familusi and Adesina (1977, 123) subsequently proposed that routine immunization with a "killed 'Salk type' vaccine," which could be combined with tetanus, diphtheria, and pertussis vaccines, should be carried out at health clinics and hospitals. In any event, these discussions were unresolved because of the political instability associated with the Nigerian Civil War (1967–70) and its aftermath and the focus on the smallpox eradication campaign, which began in 1967.

The Smallpox Eradication Campaign, 1967–70

After Nigeria became an independent state in 1960, an attempted coup by military officers in 1966 and the subsequent move by Eastern Region leaders to secede led to civil war in May 1967. This would seem to have been a particularly inopportune time for beginning an eradication campaign, yet through the cooperation of political leaders on both sides of the confrontation, approximately 68,727,000 people were immunized within a period of six years. While vaccinations were carried out in the Eastern Region prior to the onset of hostilities, in 1968 and 1969 both smallpox and measles vaccinations were provided there by the Red Cross and the World Council of Churches (Fenner et al. 1988, 883). Vaccination was also carried out by mass campaigns in the Western and Northern Regions; despite the use of inoculation methods such as those described by Baba of Karo, smallpox was more widely prevalent in the Northern Region in the 1960s than in the other two regions of Nigeria, mainly because of poor vaccination coverage (Fenner et al. 1988, 882).

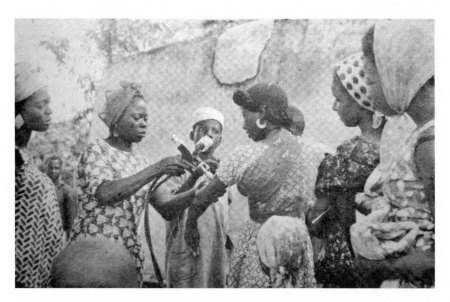

Figure 2.1. Woman giving a smallpox vaccination, using the now obsolete Ped-O-Jet injector, during the smallpox eradication campaign in the Kawo area of Kaduna, 18 September 1969. Courtesy of the *New Nigerian*.

In July 1967, vaccination for smallpox and measles began in earnest in Northern Nigeria through mass campaigns organized by edicts (with fines for noncompliance) issued by traditional rulers, much as had been proposed earlier by colonial officials through the 1917 Vaccination Ordinance. According to one program officer, "In the south, a health education programme had to reach all the people to convince them to participate in a health activity, whereas in the north, a health educator only had to convince the emirs" (Fenner et al. 1988, 884). These mass campaigns were followed up by mobile assessment teams who returned about seven to fourteen days later to evaluate coverage by inspecting people for smallpox vaccination marks (Foege, Millar, and Henderson 1975; Foster and Smith 1970;).[20] In September 1968, an effort was made to increase coverage by improving the reporting system with the assistance of CDC epidemiologists, who helped with the investigation of small outbreaks, particularly in the Northern Region, where most of the remaining cases of smallpox were occurring. The mass campaigns and follow-up coverage by mobile assessment teams continued into the next year. For example, on Monday, 15 September 1969, a notice for smallpox vaccination appeared in a local newspaper, the *New Nigerian,* which specified the locations of vaccinations centers in Kaduna (see fig. 2.1):

> SMALLPOX and measles vaccination centres have opened in Kaduna Capital Territory and vaccination exercise began in all the centres today as follows:

Today, Kawo village office, Kawo clinic, Unguwar Shanu Dispensary, Biadaraw (near small market), Unguwar Sarkin Musulmi, Unguwar Rimi Primary School, Federal Training Centre and Ketaren Banki (Baptist Pastors' School).

Tomorrow. . . . (*New Nigerian* 1969)

While many had been vaccinated during mass immunization events organized by traditional rulers in the North, those living in tiny villages and hamlets sometimes fell through the cracks. This was true of the residents of Gerere Hamlet, who were mainly seminomadic Fulani cattle-raising people. The vaccination site in their district was more than seven miles away; another site only 1½ miles away was in another district, so they were not told about immunization events. And because Gerere Hamlet residents did not feel beholden to the local traditional ruler, they did not report the initial outbreak of smallpox in January 1968. When local Native Authority health officials did hear of the outbreak and came to the village in late March, they used lanolinated vaccine that was no longer potent, so only two people were effectively immunized.[21] However, when the hamlet was revisited two weeks later, potent freeze-dried vaccine was used and the entire village was vaccinated. Ultimately there were sixty-two cases of smallpox (with one death) as a result of this outbreak, with two known cases of exportation (Pifer and Adeoye 1968).

Distance and poor roads made it difficult to identify isolated smallpox outbreaks in rural areas, as did the possibility that local authorities might try to hide such outbreaks for fear of reprisal from government officials. Thus, in March 1970, cases of smallpox were found in the northern Yoruba town of Amayo (Fenner et al. 1988, 886–87), as well as in neighboring villages and in Ilorin, the capital of Kwara State. A massive containment effort was then carried out, with house-to-house vaccination, roadblocks, and village-by-village searches (Fenner et al. 1988, 887). Although the last known case in the Amayo-Ilorin area was identified in mid-April, five subsequent cases, possibly from Ilorin, appeared in the Lagos area in April and May 1970. However, with the successful control of these cases, Nigeria was considered to be smallpox-free as of May 1970.

Comparing Smallpox and Polio in Northern Nigeria

Prior to the smallpox eradication campaign, during the first years of Nigerian independence, smallpox and polio vaccinations were carried out by state and local government medical departments, although polio vaccinations were given only upon demand. One man who worked as a health attendant in Kano during the early 1960s described the immunization and treatment of smallpox then:

The medical staff used calamine lotion on the skin and injections of M&B suspension; sometimes they did the sand treatment but I don't know how it was done. We would do these vaccinations when there was an outbreak of smallpox. Some people refused it, especially the *malamai,* who said that there must be a motive behind it. The *mai anguwai* would get people together

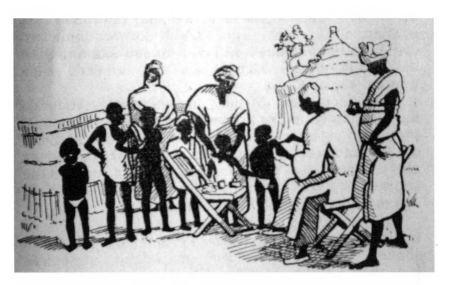

Figure 2.2. Illustration of children receiving smallpox vaccinations, from the children's book *Bala da Babiya*, by Nuhu Bamalli (1961, 45). Courtesy of Gaskiya Corporation, Zaria.

to support immunization. Sometimes they gathered at one place, and sometimes we would go house to house. Women would be in our group [to vaccinate women in seclusion]. They would put pox lymph on the arm and then cut or make small cuts with a sterile needle. The Fulani were especially the ones who were doing the old type of inoculation. The Fulani and some *malamai* were the ones resisting. But there were only a few who were resisting. (Interview, Kaduna, 27 July 2006)

As well as receiving vaccinations at local clinics and government hospitals, primary school children were vaccinated for smallpox at school during this period. They were also taught about diseases such as smallpox in health education classes. One primary school text, *Bala da Babiya: Lafiya Uwar Jiki,* written by Nuhu Bamalli, recounts stories about a husband and wife, Bala and Babiya, that emphasize the importance of hygiene for maintaining good health. In one story, Bala discovers that members of a friend's family have been stricken with small-pox (*agana*) and he works hard to make sure that everyone in the village receives smallpox vaccinations (fig. 2.2). There are no stories about polio in the book.[22]

The fact that smallpox was widely recognized as a dangerous disease while relatively few people had any experience of paralytic polio helps to explain why the Smallpox Eradication Program was able to succeed in three years in Nigeria, despite the fact that the country was at war, whereas the Polio Eradication Initiative is still ongoing there after more than ten years. Aside from differences in the perceived dangers associated with these two diseases, polio vaccination and identification faced particular logistical problems; demographic and political factors also contributed to the difficulties facing the Polio Eradication Initiative. For example, smallpox vaccination leaves a scar, clearly indicating whether an individual has received the single required dose. But the four-dose course of oral polio vaccine leaves no mark, and health cards were not used in the campaign. Thus, health workers gave multiple doses to ensure coverage. The extent of small-pox outbreaks was also clearer because of the telltale pox marks, while a single identified case of paralytic polio suggested that there were an unknown number of additional, asymptomatic polio cases. Furthermore, the large population in-creases documented by national census figures from 1963 to 2007 suggest large increases in the number of children under five who needed to receive repeated doses of oral polio vaccine. However, it was not population increase or the diffi-culties of organizing a mass polio immunization program that were mentioned by people who were asked to compare the two campaigns. Rather, they cited in-creased disillusionment with the Nigerian state as the primary reason why the Polio Eradication Initiative was considered suspect.

A cursory reading of newspapers from the late 1960s conveys a sense of the sources of this disillusionment. For even as the country was divided by civil war, newspaper stories covered the opening of new textile mills and university pro-grams, as well as the campaign to eradicate smallpox. In 1967, there was a sense of optimism that Nigeria was on the path to becoming a modern, industrialized nation. This picture contrasts with the news in 2007: stories of plant closings— the last large textile mill in Kaduna was closed in November 2007, putting four thousand people out of work (Babadoko 2007a)—of continued power shortages (Hallah 2008), and of politicians' excesses (Gulloma 2008). These failures of in-dustry, infrastructure, and political leadership have contributed to people's sense that their government has failed them. Several people mentioned distrust of the current government as a reason for suspecting the motives of those supporting the Polio Eradication Initiative, when they had not been suspicious of smallpox eradication efforts:

> Civilization [*zamani*, modernity] is just too much and people are suspicious. In those days the leaders were good but now, they are seen as immoral and worse. (Interview, Kaduna, 27 July 2006)

> People had more trust in the government then, and would do what govern-ment asked, they believed what it said. Whereas now, no one believes what government says. For example, in one small village in Giwa Local Government—when I asked people about what government does, they said, "What government?" It's only through the radio that they know anything about their government. I myself don't trust the government as an educated person—so what would villagers think? (Interview, Samaru, 8 August 2007)

People's suspicions about the polio eradication campaign have been fostered by a sense that their world has been "spoiled" by a government that cannot be trusted and by "too much civilization," too many changes to what they conceive of as the moral Hausa Muslim community in Northern Nigeria. However, this is not to say that everyone who experienced the smallpox campaign remembers it in a favorable light. One *malam* living in Zaria City explained,

> I remember the time when they were giving smallpox vaccination. People used to run away when they would see *bature* [Europeans] and they would be afraid. Polio [immunization] is better because they are Nigerians doing it and people are not afraid. (Interview, Zaria City, 25 July 2006)

Nor were earlier government health initiatives always trusted, as archival documents and more recent reports make clear. Nonetheless, the deterioration of public infrastructure in general and health services in particular during the 1990s, as well as the lack of government oversight of foreign drug trials, such as the Trovan trials in Kano during the 1996 cerebrospinal meningitis epidemic, have reinforced suspicions that the federal government and its officials are not to be trusted (Obadare 2005). This distrust, along with logistical difficulties specific to the epidemiology of polio and larger infrastructural impediments, has hampered efforts to eradicate this disease thirty-eight years after the last case of smallpox was seen in Nigeria.

✳ ✳ ✳

By examining the historical trajectories of smallpox and polio in Northern Nigeria, one gets a sense of the distinctive frames of these two diseases as well as of how local explanations of them have changed through time and circumstance. Presently, smallpox (*agana*) is barely remembered except by older people who experienced its ravages during the first half of the twentieth century. Some younger people who were not yet born at the time of the Smallpox Eradication Program do not even know the word *agana* or what the disease entailed. In effect, smallpox has been reclassified as a disease that no longer exists, except in books and on the pock-marked faces of the elderly.

Similarly, many younger people do not know that the Hausa name for poliomyelitis, Shan Inna, refers to the lame, blood-drinking *bori* spirit Inna. Indeed, they may use the term "polio," which is sometimes used in radio and television announcements promoting the recent polio eradication campaign. Shan Inna, an affliction associated with paralysis and formerly treated by *bori* spirit devotees using possession dances, sacrifices, and herbal medicines, has been reconceptualized by many Northern Nigerians as polio, which cannot be cured but may be prevented by immunization. But this reframing has not changed their belief that the disease is relatively unimportant for them. This belief is similar to that held by British colonial health officers in Nigeria before the late 1940s but differs considerably from those held by international and national health officials in later years. For the British, polio was of little concern until the late 1940s and 1950s, when expatriate colonial officials, staff, and their families who had not acquired immunity through environmental exposure as infants contracted severe cases of paralytic polio in Nigeria. Though recommendations were made that the expatriate community be immunized with the newly developed Salk vaccine in the late 1950s, immunization was not recommended for Nigerians. With Independence in 1960, polio vaccine was available on request, although polio vaccination was not a priority until it was promoted, first as part of the Expanded Programme on Immunisation, which began in Nigeria in the 1980s, and then in the Polio Eradication Initiative. Polio, initially classified as a nonthreatening endemic disease to which most Nigerians acquired immunity through environmental exposure, was reclassified as a dangerous disease that threatened populations both in Nigeria and as far away as Indonesia (Dyer 2005), and that needed to be prevented through vaccination. Thus, while Northern Nigerians' and health officials' assessments of the seriousness of polio coincided during the colonial era, later Western beliefs about the importance of polio and its eradication differs considerably from those of many Northern Nigerians.

A historical examination of smallpox during the precolonial, colonial, and Independence periods in Northern Nigeria helps to explain the problems which the recent initiative has met, since some of the problems faced in past health campaigns have reappeared. For instance, smallpox immunization efforts in colonial Northern Nigeria were faced with immense challenges—poor roads, lack of trained staff, limited numbers of health centers, and an ineffective monitoring and reporting system. Similarly, some of the solutions—such as offering a range of medical treatments, as was done during the colonial smallpox campaigns described for the Tukur area in Taraba State—have been repeated in the recent Immunization Plus Days. When one considers the historical trajectories of these two diseases, the differences in the ways that they have been reframed by Northern Nigerians and by those from the West provide another perspective from which to understand experiences of the Polio Eradication Initiative.

3. Politics and Polio in Nigeria

If we vaccinate our children we are protecting their health. We should forever protect our neighborhoods, cities, and nation from diseases such as polio.

—Radio advertisement for the Polio Eradication Initiative

From day one in 1996 when Nigeria started witnessing selective eradication of one immunisable disease, the stakeholders (Federal Ministry of Health, NPI, UNICEF, WHO, and Rotary International) . . . are shying away from the only reason that brought about the skepticism. In simple language *polio is not a priority disease of children in Nigeria.*

—Magashi, "Dr. Murzi, UNICEF and polio in Nigeria"

Our national health system has become the greatest obstacle to achieving health for all Nigerians.

—Tomori, *Politics and Disease Control in Nigeria*

Following the successful eradication of smallpox, the World Health Assembly voted in 1988 to implement a campaign to eradicate poliomyelitis by the end of the year 2000 (WHA 1988a). While some public health specialists were skeptical about the possibility of accomplishing this goal because of the difficulty of identifying asymptomatic cases of wild poliovirus and of distinguishing wild poliovirus from other enteroviruses (Yekutiel 1980, 153), developments in genetic sequencing of viruses in fecal samples from children with acute flaccid paralysis have improved the identification of virus strains, allowing health personnel to identify continuing sources of infection. Yet concerns about the logistical difficulties of providing multiple doses of the oral polio vaccine and the necessary continued monitoring and testing of fecal samples have led others to question continuing the eradication campaign (Arita, Nakane, and Fenner 2006; Reynolds 2007; Roberts 2006; see also Steinglass's response to Dobriansky et al. 2007). While health workers have faced some of the same obstacles that arose during the Smallpox Eradication Program, including poor basic infrastructure, low levels of immunization, and transportation problems, mainly it has been political factors which have confounded the successful conclusion of the Polio Eradication Initiative in Nigeria.

Nonetheless, health officials and workers associated with the Polio Eradication Initiative are optimistic (Dobriansky et al. 2007; Heymann and Aylward 2004; Pallansch and Sandhu 2006). In Northern Nigeria, there is cause for both optimism and skepticism. After organizational changes in the National

Programme on Immunization and the implementation of Immunization Plus Days in 2006, confirmed cases of wild poliovirus declined significantly in 2007, although they increased again in 2008 (WHO 2009; see table 1.1). These recent increases may be attributed to leadership problems at the federal level, which are reflected in basic infrastructural declines, economic constraints which limited the health incentives offered during National Immunization Days, and outbreaks of cerebrospinal meningitis in early 2009,[1] all of which fostered public distrust of government health initiatives.

These problems may be seen more clearly through an examination of the background of the Polio Eradication Initiative in Northern Nigeria, beginning with the introduction of the Expanded Programme on Immunisation in 1979 and continuing with its reorganization as the National Programme on Immunization in the mid-1990s. This Programme, which was responsible for the running of the Polio Eradication Initiative, was affected by politics from its inception. Political factors were reflected in its organization and leadership, its conduct of the campaign, and its later restructuring under the National Primary Health Care Development Agency (NPHCDA) in 2006. Politics was also a factor in the temporary ban on polio immunization in several Northern Nigerian states in 2003. These political factors influenced Northern Nigerian parents' experiences and acceptance of the polio campaign. In Zaria, the debate over the safety of the polio vaccine in 2003 reinforced the convictions of some that it was unsafe. Although some parents and Islamic teachers continued to question its safety, the focus on community participation and the provision of health incentives during Immunization Plus Days, instituted in May 2006, contributed to other parents' acceptance of it, as is reflected in the decline in polio cases in 2007. The increase in 2008 suggests that although many Muslim Northern Nigerians who initially protested against polio eradication have come to accept the polio campaign, a continuing sense of political insecurity complicates the problems facing the Polio Eradication Initiative.

Implementing the Polio Eradication Initiative in Nigeria

At the forty-first meeting of the World Health Assembly, in 1988, member states were directed to work to eradicate poliomyelitis, with the understanding "that achievement of the goal will depend on the political will of countries and on the investment of adequate human and financial resources" (WHA 1988b). In Nigeria, both political will and the levels of human and financial resources invested have waxed and waned. Several national and international organizations have supported the Polio Eradication Initiative, including the Nigerian Federal Ministry of Health, the National Programme on Immunization, UN agencies such as WHO and UNICEF, U.S.-based agencies and nongovernmental organizations (NGOs) including the Centers for Disease Control and Prevention–Atlanta, USAID, and the Gates Foundation, and the European Union, the World Bank, and Rotary International. It is estimated that from the beginning of 1985 to July 2007, individual countries, international nongovernmental agencies, and nonprofit organizations spent approximately US$5.2 billion worldwide on the Polio Eradication Initiative (WHO 2007a). However, in Nigeria, the decline in routine childhood immunization, which had been introduced though the UNICEF program known as the Expanded Programme on Immunisation, complicated polio eradication efforts. The difficulty in carrying out the Initiative, as well as in revitalizing routine immunization, reflects the shifting political and economic fortunes of primary health care there.

The Expanded Programme on Immunisation in Nigeria

The Expanded Programme on Immunisation began in Nigeria in 1979, shortly after the eradication of smallpox was certified. The World Health Organization had instituted this program in 1974, with the goal of providing vaccines for diphtheria, pertussis, tetanus, measles, polio, and tuberculosis to more than 80 percent of children worldwide (Ekanem 1988). Health officials sought to reach a level of coverage high enough to provide "herd immunity" (Henderson 1999, S55), so that even children who were not immunized would be protected from these childhood diseases. The goal of this ambitious program was attained in some countries, particularly those with well-developed health infrastructures and trained personnel. However, in Nigeria, infrastructural, political, and economic problems hampered routine immunization. Indeed, immunization levels for the early 1980s were low, ranging from 5 to 10 percent (Federal Ministry of Health, Nigeria 1991, 3). These low levels were partly due to political and economic instability during the period from 1979 to 1985, when Nigerians elected a civilian president and subsequently experienced two military coups. In 1985 General Ibrahim Babangida, anxious to gain international approval for his government, appointed Professor Olikoye Ransome-Kuti as minister of health. It was Ransome-Kuti who established a program of primary health care centers throughout the country where vaccines were made widely available (Olatimehin 1988, 3). In March 1988, the first phase of a national immunization exercise was held at primary health care centers. Free vaccines were distributed, although nationwide only 50 percent of children under two years old were immunized. In 1989, Ransome-Kuti pledged to achieve 80 percent coverage by December 1990 (Orere 1989, 20), in line with the UNICEF goal of universal childhood immunization for vaccine-preventable diseases of early childhood. In Nigeria, this level of immunization against tuberculosis, using the Bacillus Calmette-Guérin vaccine, was in fact achieved (National Planning Commission and UNICEF 2001, 84).

The year 1990 is considered to be the high point of national immunization coverage. However, on 30 June 1990, responsibility for primary health care services was transferred to the local governments as part of a structural adjustment program initiated by the International Monetary Fund, which required the federal government to curtail spending on social services (Anonymous 1990), and in 1991, states were required to purchase their own vaccines (A. Umar 1989, 24). Since vaccines used during the Expanded Programme on Immunisation drive in 1990 were provided by UNICEF and other NGOs via the federal government without charge to local governments, when federal responsibility for primary health care services was transferred to local governments the availability of vaccines drastically declined, as one Ahmadu Bello University professor explained:

> Now, when that happened there was now almost zero coverage, because the chairman, the local government did not take it seriously because they do not want to spend money there. And of course, the truth of the matter was that they were not awarding the contract or procurement. So there was no money forthcoming along that [road] and they didn't want to spend their money. (Interview, Zaria, 20 July 2005)

Subsequently, the system of routine immunization through primary health care clinics and hospitals in local government areas broke down.[2] Overall immunization levels, as represented by diphtheria, pertussis, and tetanus (DPT3) coverage, declined, and by 1993, government data indicated that they had sunk to around 30 percent (FBA Health Systems Analysts 2005, 3). This decline in immunization levels, including complete sequences of polio vaccination, may be seen in a comparison of data from the 1990 and 1999 Nigerian Demographic and Health Surveys (Bonu, Rani, and Razum 2004, 333; see also National Population Commission and ORC Macro 2004). A sense of this decline is more dramatically represented in a 1996 issue of the national news magazine *Newswatch:*

> Nothing perhaps exhibits the poor state of things like the primary health care programme. Olikoye Ransome-Kuti who was health minister between 1985 and 1992 did a lot to attract foreign aid for the programme which aims to immunize children against childhood communicable diseases, like measles, polio, tetanus, whooping cough and tuberculosis. . . .
> Oladunmi Alabi's three children benefited from the programme. When Alabi had her fourth baby last March [1996] she thought she would just walk into the Isolo General Hospital to immunize her. She was directed to the primary health centre near by. There she ran into other nursing mothers waiting to get their babies immunized.
> "I didn't know things have changed so drastically," she told *Newswatch* adding, "I had to go three times before I could get the first immunization for my daughter." (Anonymous 1996, 10)

Later that year, UNICEF approved a plan to provide US$82 million to Nigeria to improve this situation. A four-year program was to provide vaccines and medicines for early childhood diseases (Ugwu 1996, 31), although vaccine provision has remained a problem (NPHCDA 2007, 9). In the same year, a national program established to replace the Expanded Programme on Immunisation was also launched.

The Reorganization of the Expanded Programme on Immunisation as the National Programme on Immunization

The early 1990s saw not just a shift from federal to local responsibility for immunization but also considerable political uncertainty due to electioneering and the subsequent annulment of the national presidential election in June 1993. Nationwide strikes (in which health workers participated) helped to force President Babangida's resignation in August, which was followed by a three-month interim presidency and a bloodless coup led by General Sani Abacha in November 1993.

With the change in national leadership, there was political interest in revitalizing the national immunization program. In July 1995, the Expanded Programme on Immunisation was renamed the National Programme on Immunization, in order to stress national responsibility for immunization (Alabi 1995; interview, Kaduna, 7 September 2005). In 1996, the National Programme on Immunization was formally launched as part of the Family Support Programme, a project run by the first lady, Miriam Abacha. In August 1997, the NPI's legal mandate was set forth in Decree No. 12 of 1997, which created the National Programme on Immunization as a separate parastatal (FBA Health Systems Analysts 2005; interview, Kaduna, 7 September 2005), meaning that it operated as an independent agency whose director was appointed by and responsible to the Nigerian head of state.[3] However, in practice its staff worked closely with the Federal Ministry of Health and with international agencies and groups such as WHO, UNICEF, and Rotary International.

One year after the National Programme on Immunization was launched, it came under the direction of Dr. Dere Awosika, a pharmacist who was the daughter of Festus Okotie-Eboh, the first minister of finance (Benjamin 2005). She continued in this position under two successive presidents, until she was forced to resign in December 2005. In 2007 the Programme was merged with another parastatal, the NPHCDA, under the Ministry of Health. During its tenure, the National Programme on Immunization was responsible for importing vaccines and distributing them to cold-store centers throughout the country. It was also responsible for promoting immunization in Nigeria, which included distributing oral polio vaccine and promoting the Polio Eradication Initiative.

Dynamics of Acceptance and Rejection of the Polio Eradication Initiative

The Polio Eradication Initiative began in Nigeria in 1996, although not all states participated in the first round of immunizations (*Guardian* 1997, 3). Since routine immunization had declined during the 1990s, National Programme on Immunization officials organized National Immunization Days, aiming to initiate a mass immunization program for polio rather than relying on mothers bringing their children in for immunization at clinics and hospitals. This entailed hiring and training vaccination team members as well as distributing cold chain equipment and vaccine. They also needed to establish a system for monitoring the wild poliovirus: children with acute flaccid paralysis (in one or more limbs) had to be identified and stool specimens from them collected and transported (CDC 2005, 873). The results of these early efforts were mixed, as

Table 3.1. National Immunization, Sub-National Immunization, and "Mop-Up" Days, Ghana and Nigeria, 2001–2009[1]

		2001	2002	2003	2004	2005	2006	2007	2008	2009
GHANA										
	NIDs (n)	2^2	—	1^4	4^5	3^6	1	1	1	4^7
	SNIDS (n)	2	2^3	2	—	—	—	—	1	—
	Mop-up (n)	—	—	1	—	—	—	—	—	—
	TOTAL	4	2	4	4	3	1	1	2	4
NIGERIA										
	NIDs (n)	4	3	—	5	4	2	3	2	4
	SNIDS (n)	1	2	7	2	2	6	9	11	11
	Mop-up (n)	—	3	4	—	—	2	5	2	—
	TOTAL	5	8	11	7	6	10	17	15	15

Notes:

1. Schedule from January 2001 to June 2009.
2. Both NIDs in Ghana in 2001 were part of synchronized National Immunization Days held in Nigeria, Niger, Benin, Burkina Faso, and Togo.
3. Both SNIDs in Ghana in 2002 were part of synchronized National Immunization Days held in Nigeria, Niger, Benin, Burkina Faso, and Togo.
4. The NID in Ghana in 2003 was part of synchronized National Immunization Days held in Niger, Benin, Burkina Faso, and Togo; in Nigeria an SNID was held.
5. All four NIDs in Ghana in 2004 were part of synchronized National Immunization Days held in Nigeria, Niger, Benin, Burkina Faso, and Togo.
6. All three NIDS in Ghana in 2005 were part of synchronized National Immunization Days held in Nigeria, Niger, Benin, and Burkina Faso.
7. Ghana, Nigeria, Niger, Benin, Burkina Faso, and Togo held synchronized National Immunization Days in summer 2009 to address outbreaks.

Source: WHO, Supplementary Immunization Activities Calendar, http://www.who.int/ immunization_monitoring/en/globalsummary/siacalendar/padvancedsia.cfm, accessed 13 December 2009.

evidenced by the large percentages of cases of acute flaccid paralysis which were confirmed as caused by wild poliovirus (65 percent in 2000) and by the low levels of stool sample viability (36 percent in the same year). It was not until 2001 that more than 40 percent of the stool specimens sent for laboratory testing were viable (see table 1.1).

When the initial goal of global polio eradication by the end of the year 2000 was not met,[4] WHO officials extended the deadline to 2005 (WHO 2000) and immunization activities in Nigeria increased. Four National Immunization Days in 2001 and three in 2002 (WHO 2007b) were supplemented by Sub-National Immunization Days, during which efforts were directed toward states and local government areas where cases of acute flaccid paralysis continued to appear and where immunization coverage was low. During three "mop-up" days in 2002, health workers focused on specific wards and neighborhoods to improve vaccination levels (table 3.1). All children under the age of five were given oral polio vaccine, regardless of whether they had received earlier doses, in order to ensure universal coverage, since cards recording vaccination histories were not used.

During this period of increased vaccination open resistance to the Polio Eradication Initiative emerged in Northern Nigeria, with parents refusing to allow health workers to enter their homes or vaccinate their children, and sometimes physically and verbally abusing health workers. These parents' distrust of and resistance to the campaign, expressed in rumors that the polio vaccine was contaminated with contraceptive substances or HIV-AIDS, was reinforced in 2003 when the safety of the oral polio vaccine was questioned by a range of individuals in Northern Nigeria, including medical doctors, university professors, and Muslim scholars, as well as politicians.[5]

Testing Oral Polio Vaccine Safety

In July 2003, increasing suspicions about the Polio Eradication Initiative and about the safety of the polio vaccine led the head of the Supreme Council for Shari'a (Muslim law) to call for a suspension of polio vaccination (Babadoko 2003).[6] The governor of Kano State, Ibrahim Shekarau, set up a technical committee to investigate polio vaccine safety in October 2003 and announced that polio vaccination in Kano State would be halted until tests could be conducted to confirm vaccine safety (Ibrahim 2003; Obadare 2005; Renne 2006; Yahya 2007). Kano is the most populous state of Northern Nigeria.

The events in Kano State contributed to a cascade of events, widely reported in the news media, which impeded the implementation of the polio campaign in Northern Nigeria. In fall 2003, the Kaduna State government set up a committee to test the polio vaccine for contaminants, with tests carried out at Ahmadu Bello University Teaching Hospital in Zaria and at the National Hospital in Abuja (G. Muhammad 2003). Officials from the National Programme on Immunization, the Ministry of Health, and the World Health Organization countered that the Kaduna State tests needed to be duplicated for confirmation. The Federal Ministry of Health subsequently organized a team which went to test the vaccine in South Africa (G. Muhammad 2003, 1–2), while Jama'atu Nasril Islam, the umbrella organization for Muslims in Northern Nigeria, sent a team of its own experts to test the vaccine in Indian labs. On 23 December 2003, the minister of health, Professor Eyitayo Lambo, announced that the "Oral Polio Vaccine (OPV) used in Nigeria for immunisation, . . . had been found to be safe and free of antifertility agents and HIV" (Okpani 2003b). However, one month later, the Jama'atu Nasril Islam team, which included two members of the Faculty of Pharmaceutical Sciences at Ahmadu Bello University, officially announced that they found the polio vaccine to be contaminated (Babadoko and Kazaure 2004, 1–2).[7]

These contradictory findings contributed to the refusal by the governor of Kano State to use vaccines provided by WHO (*Weekly Trust* 2003, 1; Kazaure 2004) and to allow the resumption of the polio campaign there. However, after additional tests were jointly carried out by Ministry of Health and Jama'atu Nasril Islam experts (Okpani 2003b), Alhaji Muhammadu Maccido, the Sultan of Sokoto and head of the Muslim community in Nigeria, announced on 17 March 2004, "Oral polio vaccine is safe" (*Daily Trust* 2004b), and the announcement was publicized by a photograph of his giving a child oral polio vaccine in a 2004 calendar sponsored by UNICEF. This endorsement did not convince everyone, although the situation was eventually remedied by the importation of polio vaccines from Indonesia, announced by the Kano State commissioner of health on 17 May 2004 (*Daily Trust* 2004a). After discussing the situation with officials and religious leaders in Kano, the governor agreed to resume polio vaccinations in Kano on 29 July 2004 (Musa 2004). He had his own children publicly vaccinated, and the Emir of Kano, Alhaji Ado Bayero, gave his approval of the Polio Eradication Initiative.

Although the ban was lifted, many confirmed cases of polio were reported in subsequent years, particularly in Kano State (Obadare 2005; Renne 2006; Yahya 2007). Many parents in Kano and elsewhere in the North continued to refuse having health workers immunize their children. This resistance also reflected other recent events, particularly in Kano, where officials of the Federal Ministry of Health had failed to protect people during the drug trial of the antibiotic Trovan, which—like polio vaccine—had been distributed free of charge during the 1996 cerebrospinal meningitis epidemic (Obadare 2005; Olusanya 2004; see chapter 7). Some parents were genuinely afraid to have their children vaccinated, in part because of distrust of the federal government. Others questioned the program's exclusive focus on polio immunization and wondered why they were asked to allow their children to be repeatedly immunized on multiple National Immunization Day rounds. Consequently in 2008, Kano State had the largest number of cases of wild poliovirus in Nigeria (*Nation* 2008).

The Polio Eradication Initiative in Zaria

It is against this backdrop of a decline in primary health care, public distrust of polio eradication efforts, and federal politics that polio immunization took place in Zaria, in northern Kaduna State. The town of Zaria is the site of the old Hausa Emirate of Zazzau, which is presided over by the current Emir of Zaria, Alhaji Shehu Idris. While not as large as the megacity of Kano, it is famous for trade and for its educational institutions, including several Islamic schools and the oldest tertiary institution in Northern Nigeria, Ahmadu Bello University, which has a well-established teaching hospital. Indeed, several members of its faculty had been involved in the debates over the safety of the oral polio vaccine. While the general public in Zaria might not have followed all the intricacies of their arguments, they nonetheless would have heard about these discussions through radio programs, at social functions, at mosques, and in schools. For some, the test results and the approval given by the Sultan of Sokoto and Jama'atu Nasril Islam settled the controversy, as one Zaria City woman explained:

The reason why I accepted the polio vaccine—it is said that prevention is better than cure. You say you would like to have it because you are afraid the disease will catch you. To avoid that you will take the vaccine. When you immunize [a child], even if the disease catches the child, it will not catch them very well. And another reason; I have seen parents taking their children for vaccination so it makes me accept it. I used to encourage my relatives about the vaccine. . . . When you have seen it on TV and heard it on the radio all the time, even those who do not agree with it, later they will agree. Because they will see children given the vaccine; nothing happened to them. (Interview, Zaria City, 6 July 2005)

Yet for others, the controversy simply reinforced what they already feared about the polio vaccine, as one farmer observed:

No, I don't allow my children to have the vaccine because I don't trust the vaccine. Because they said they are going to do it free of charge. And if we go to the hospital, we have to buy medicine and it is costly there. But this one is free of charge—in the hospital, your child can die or your brother can die if you don't have money.

My children have had measles vaccine, but this polio vaccine, I won't allow it. I took them to the hospital to do the measles vaccine, they didn't come to my house. And I never took my children for any immunization except this measles vaccine. . . .

I never heard the sultan [of Sokoto] explain this polio vaccine on the radio or anything. When they come to my house, I told them I don't want them to do it for my children, and the health worker, she just went out. . . . .

If I believe in polio or go to the hospital and have medicine free of charge, like this polio, I can accept the polio vaccine. But if I have to pay for medicine in the hospital, I will not accept this one. (Interview, Samaru, September 2005)

Some parents refused the polio vaccine because they believed it was contaminated. This man, however, was opposed to a campaign which focused on a single disease and did not provide affordable primary health care for children. In other words, he did not approve of, nor would he participate in, a top-down approach to the health care of his children in which he had no say.

Thus, there were several reasons why some parents in Zaria did not bring their children to hospitals or clinics for polio immunization or allow health workers to administer the oral polio vaccine in their homes. Some distrusted the motivations of those promoting a Western health intervention and saw "Christian countries' concern to export biomedicine to all parts of Africa . . . not as a chari-table gesture but as self-interested and dangerous" (M. Last 2005, 561). Others distrusted the federal government, under President Olusegun Obasanjo, and the heads of both the Ministry of Health and the National Programme on Immunization, all of whom were southern Nigerians and whom they held responsible for the deteriorating health conditions and poorly regulated drug trials in Northern Nigeria (Obadare 2005, 280). By focusing on the eradication of polio, which many people did not see as a primary health problem for their children, and not improving primary health care—including routine provision of early childhood vaccines, which were frequently unavailable,[8] and free treatment for malaria—health officials and their international partners were, parents believed, indirectly contributing to the deaths of their children. For example, measles was considered to be a life-threatening illness in Northern Nigeria, while polio was considered to be only a minor problem. Yet before December 2005, only polio vaccine and Vitamin A supplements were available during National Immunization Days and Sub-National Immunization Days, whereas in the earlier smallpox eradication campaign measles vaccine (for control) was also administered. Consequently, public health specialists working in northeastern Nigeria noted that

> while three confirmed cases of poliomyelitis registered in Adamawa State in 2005 triggered massive resource mobilisation and action, hundreds of children dying due to measles during the same time frame did not elicit anything close to an appropriate outbreak response. . . . Sustained vaccine coverage for measles of below 40%, as in Nigeria, in an era of regular immunisation days for polio is highly disconcerting. (Schimmer and Ihekweazu 2006)

However, after the Immunization Plus Days were implemented in May 2006, measles vaccine was regularly provided as part of the polio campaign. Yet despite this and other health incentives, some parents continued to fear the effects of the oral polio vaccine on their children and to distrust the safety of immunization injections more generally. In March 1995 during a Rotary Club immunization project in Zaria City, for instance, parents became concerned about boils occurring around the site of immunization and about a loss of hearing (Renne 1996).[9] Others had heard that the attenuated live virus used in the polio vaccine can actually cause polio, and some knew that inactivated poliovirus vaccine (IPV) was being used in the West, since the topic has been discussed in the Nigerian press (*Weekly Trust* 2003). One woman whose daughter was diagnosed as having polio insisted that the child had received as many as ten doses of the vaccine. She assumed that the vaccine had caused her daughter's illness (interview, Zaria, 15 July 2005).

A House in Zaria City

While uncertainty about the safety of immunization was not uncommon in Zaria, how some parents weighed the benefits and risks of polio immunization may be seen in the actions of two mothers, each of whom had a four-year-old son, who were living in one house in Zaria City, a section of the larger city of Zaria. From the mark "SNID" (standing for Sub-National Polio Immunization Day) written near the main entryway leading into the family compound, one might be led to believe that all children under five years living in the house, including these two boys, had been vaccinated for polio. However, this was not the case. I was told that it only meant that the house had been visited by an immunization team, who were not allowed to enter.

That visit had been made in 2004. In 2006, the young boys' mothers' resistance to house-to-house immunization was countered by polio immunization teams in two ways. First, polio vaccines were administered in nursery and primary schools providing Western education (*boko*); one of the boys was attending such a school. Second, vaccinations were given at a mass immunization program in front of the Emir of Zaria's palace. The two young mothers heard of the mass immunization program from radio announcements, and Malam, the household head and father of one of the women, told them to attend. One took her son to the palace but did not stay long enough to have him immunized, because there were many women already there and she didn't have time. Furthermore, her son had been immunized in nursery school, although this had been done without her permission.[10] The other young mother took her son for immunization at the palace, where he received one of the four necessary doses of oral polio vaccine. However, she subsequently refused to allow health workers to vaccinate him when they came to the house. In both cases, their children were given oral polio drops outside of their house. Indeed, according to the mother attending the mass immunization program, the vaccine given in the house was contaminated with medicine (*magani*) that destroys their children's fertility (*yana kashe kwayoyi haihuwa*, literally, it kills the eggs of childbearing), while vaccine given in public—at school or at mass immunization programs authorized by the Emir of Zaria—was not. It seems that immunization in public venues which the women trusted imparted confidence in the vaccine, where private immunization by strangers in their homes did not.[11]

The behavior of immunization team members—who sometimes behaved inappropriately, some refusing to follow local practices such as veiling (interview, Zaria City, 31 August 2005), and some who were so young and poorly trained that they could not answer parents' questions (Yahya 2007, 195)—led parents to refuse to allow them to immunize their children. These problems were also mentioned by health officials, who noted that some team members were themselves opposed to the polio immunization program but needed a job (interview, Samaru, 8 August 2005). Maintaining a positive attitude in the face of open hostility to the campaign would be difficult under any circumstances. However, the focus on polio vaccination and failure to provide other, more relevant health treatments was to change significantly in 2006, making the jobs of immunization team members considerably easier.

Revising the Polio Eradication Initiative

Health workers associated with the National Programme on Immunization, WHO, and UNICEF attempted to meet the new deadline of December 2005 for global polio eradication through additional house-to-house vaccination exercises in Zaria. During these visits, immunization teams worked in groups of six (and at times, up to eight)—two recorders, two vaccinators, a crowd-controller, and a ward head—along with a supervisor. One woman who worked on a team described the etiquette of entering a house and seeking permission to vaccinate:

> If I enter a house, I will do *salama alaikum* [a greeting] to them as Hausa people are doing. I will tell them we came to do polio vaccine to immunize

their children. [I will tell them that] there is a need to eradicate this disease in Nigeria—just like smallpox was eradicated. I will ask them if any of their children have *sanyi kafa,* cold legs [pain or paralysis in their legs], or if they have high fever. We will tell them the symptoms and if they don't have the symptoms, then I will ask them to bring the children so we can look and see. Some brought their children and some did not. (Interview, Zaria City, 31 August 2005)

When parents agreed to have their children vaccinated, the children's thumbs were stained with gentian violet. On leaving the house, a team member would mark the doorway to show that the house had been visited and whether vaccine was administered or not.

As has been mentioned, some parents saw the appearance of immunizing teams at their homes as an intrusive imposition which they refused to accept. One mother explained,

There was a time I nearly slapped one of those polio workers who came to the house. She [told] me to bring the children, but I said I didn't like the polio vaccine and refused. She began talking and tried to convince me. But I nearly slapped her and asked her to go. (Interview, Zaria City, August 2005)[12]

However, when the newly structured Immunization Plus Days were introduced in mid-2006 (plate 1), immunization workers in Zaria City saw less resistance to polio vaccination and were optimistic that they might be able to complete their work:

I have experienced a lot, because there are a lot of problems. Because most [of] the people rejected it but now some are receptive. . . . Now most of the people are accepting, they have been enlightened. . . . Maybe this year we will finish it because some of the people who resisted before are accepting it now. (Interview, Zaria City, 25 July 2006)

This acceptance reflected the shift from merely providing polio vaccine and Vitamin A to also distributing insecticide-treated bednets, deworming medicines, and soap, as well as a range of vaccines including measles vaccine, at fixed posts. These "health incentives" had a positive impact, as one official explained:

Those who didn't want their children to have the vaccine before, they come out now to get the bednets and allow their children to take vaccine. And . . . we are doing injections for diphtheria, pertussis, and measles, [and] tetanus toxoid for pregnant women, also yellow fever. . . . Those six [health workers] who are going house to house, they are the ones telling the people to take their children to the fixed post. They will tell them the type of injection [they need] and that they should take their children. (Interview, Zaria City, 2 August 2007)

Mothers with one or two children who had health cards that showed they had received the full series of polio, diphtheria-pertussis-tetanus toxoid, and measles vaccinations were given one bednet, while those with three or more were given two nets. This strategy was not without complications, as health workers discovered. In a reversal of the earlier rejection of vaccination, some mothers took their children to receive multiple doses at different sites, or loaned them to other women so they could get bednets too. The demand for bednets was so great that supplies ran out.[13] Consequently, health workers scrutinized cards more closely and sought to carefully identify children. While it is not clear precisely how these changes influenced Zaria City parents' decisions to allow their children to be immunized, the provision of insecticide-treated bednets was strongly supported by one woman:

> Really, it is a good thing they are doing. If they are taking bednets house to house, it will be good because some, they don't know they are distributing the bednet in the hospital. I will agree for the polio people to do polio for my child because I need the bednet. (Interview, Zaria City, August 2006)

The success of Immunization Plus Days, along with other programs instituted in 2006, contributed to the decline in confirmed cases of wild poliovirus in Kaduna State in 2006 and 2007. This shift in immunization policy reflected another change, that of the leadership of the National Programme on Immunization in December 2005.

Changes in the Polio Eradication Initiative and Attention to Local Concerns

In November 2005, the Northern Nigerian newspaper *The Daily Trust* published an article criticizing the leadership of the director of the National Programme on Immunization, Dr. Dere Awosika, who was a political appointee by the Abacha administration. The author reported that the World Bank country director had written that unless the National Programme on Immunization improved its management of immunization, the World Bank would discontinue its support for immunization in Nigeria (Haruna 2005). This public criticism followed several years of discontent with the workings of the National Programme on Immunization among foreign donors.[14] In December 2005 Dr. Awosika submitted her resignation, and in January 2006 the newly appointed acting director, Dr. Edugie Abebe, immediately set about revamping the Programme (Gulloma 2006, 39). The National Immunization Days, with their focus on polio vaccination, were reorganized as the Immunization Plus Days program in May 2006 (WHA 2007), and program practices were changed in other ways to take account of local perspectives.

In March 2006, after the Expert Review Committee meeting (which consisted of officials from the National Programme on Immunization and the Ministry of Health, along with others from WHO, CDC, and USAID), health officials introduced the Community Participation for Action in the Social Sector (COMPASS) polio program, which focused on polio immunization in the six states in Northern Nigeria—Jigawa, Kaduna, Katsina, Kebbi, Sokoto, and Zamfara—where polio was endemic.[15] One of the first steps taken by COMPASS-Polio in Kaduna State was to establish partnerships with local community groups, including Polio Victims Trust Associations (organizations established in several Northern Nigerian states for people disabled by polio) and the Federation of Muslim Women's Associations in Nigeria. Members of these groups were incorporated in various ways into Immunization Plus Days (Renne 2009). For example, members of the Polio Victims Trust Association sometimes accompanied immunization teams, as one member explained:

> We will go with them to the *mai anguwar* [neighborhood head] and will explain to him about the polio program and that they want to give the polio medicine to their children under five years. If I meet a person who doesn't agree to immunize their children, I will talk to them, and some will bring their children and some will not agree. We did it in Zaria City—the first set we did were about thirty. We went to different quarters—the first time they took Anguwar Jumma for five days and the second time, Anguwar Kwarbai. Within those days, there was only one day in which people refused to accept us. On the other days, people brought their children. (Interview, Yakasai, 3 August 2006)

COMPASS personnel also met with political and religious leaders in communities where resistance to the Polio Eradication Initiative was high in order to identify people who had influence with local people. These community leaders would then work together to talk with recalcitrant parents in their villages, and some also went to other communities as part of a health education campaign. In addition, community drama was used as a form of communication to convey information and dispel misconceptions about the oral polio vaccine (plate 2). This community dialogue, as well as the institution of extra Immunization Plus Days (in which COMPASS was also involved) and the mass polio immunization programs sponsored by traditional political leaders such as the Emir of Zaria, significantly reduced the number of confirmed cases of wild poliovirus reported in Kaduna State in 2007. By 1 July 2007, there were only four, as compared with forty wild poliovirus cases in the first six months of 2006 (WHO Kaduna 2006, 2007b).

While limited funds and a universal protocol may militate against tailoring global eradication efforts to address local considerations, the apparent success of these revised immunization programs, along with the advocacy of trusted community leaders in Zaria, supports what one community leader involved in immunization efforts said about the conduct of national public health campaigns:

> It helps because we talked to them, and I will use this opportunity to give government some advice if they are going to do something like polio in the future. They need to contact big people because we live among them, we used

to help them, and if we talk to them, they will accept. But if they use *'yan boko* [those who are like Westerners; literally, sons of Western education], they will not accept because they don't like *'yan boko*. But big people in the town, they are always in the town and they take good care of them—that would help very much. But if they didn't use the big people, if the government comes with something—even if it is very good—most people will not accept. (Interview, Zaria City, 3 August 2006)

Accepting and Protesting Polio and the Political Impediments to Immunization

When the Expert Review Committee on Polio Eradication and Routine Immunization in Nigeria met in Abuja in November 2007 to assess the year's activities and plan for the upcoming year, its members noted that "as of 8 November 2007, a total of 225 cases of paralytic poliomyelitis (polio) due to wild poliovirus have been confirmed in 23 states, compared with 992 cases in 18 states during the same period in 2006" (NPHCDA 2007, 4). This striking decline in cases was attributed to the improved management of the polio campaign, especially the implementation of Immunization Plus Days, along with increased community involvement in areas with low rates of immunization and the expansion of the Polio Eradication Initiative to attend to a wider range of childhood health problems. These changes had made parents more willing to have their children immunized. The success of the distribution of insecticide-treated bednets in improving polio immunization rates suggests that when Western commodities are wanted, rumors that such commodities are contaminated with contraceptives do not arise. Indeed, when one woman who had received a bednet at a local antenatal clinic was explicitly asked about its treatment with insecticide, she replied,

The bednet is very good. And they said that the ones they are using have medicine, the mosquito cannot enter the bednet or even come near. I like everything about bednets, there is nothing about them that I don't like. Even when there is heat I use it because there is mosquito. (Interview, Zaria City, July 2006)

Women want to protect their children from malaria, and a bednet is a powerful incentive to have them vaccinated.

Nonetheless, some parents remain unconvinced that the oral polio vaccine is safe. This view is supported by Islamic teachers in Zaria City, who in the past have discouraged mothers from allowing their children to be vaccinated. One woman whose daughter had contracted polio explained, "In Islamiyya school, they [teachers] would tell people not to give their children the vaccine because there is something bad in it. It is because of this, that here in Locus [her neighborhood], in one in every five houses, you will find people who refuse to immunize their children" (interview, Zaria City, 9 August 2005). Many Islamiyya teachers in Zaria City still hold this position. They prefer, as one put it, to place their faith in prayers to Allah, who will provide the protection they need. According to him, Zaria City mothers who now take their children for immunization have been misled by the provision of bednets and other health incentives.

The provision of free, improved primary health care services may convince many, but not all, parents to allow their children to be vaccinated, although immunization has had a mixed reception in Zaria. When there is an imminent danger, immunization is viewed as beneficial; during the 1996 cerebrospinal meningitis epidemic there was a high demand for vaccine (Ejembi, Renne, and Adamu 1998). However, routine immunization has been seen by some Zaria residents as unnecessary or possibly even dangerous for healthy infants and children. Recent data indicates that routine immunization levels in Kaduna State from January to June 2007 are quite low in some local government areas, which suggests that fears about vaccinating children persist.

However, Northern Nigerian parents' fears about immunization reflect another aspect of the Polio Eradication Initiative and primary health care. While the implementation of National Immunization Days has been improved, with measles vaccines, Vitamin A tablets, and paracetamol being provided in 2008 and 2009, continuing leadership changes in the Ministry of Health have undermined the consistent running of these programs. With the election of a new president, Umaru Yar'Adua, in 2007, the National Programme on Immunization was merged into the National Primary Health Care Development Agency, which was directed by Mrs. Titilola Koleoso-Adelekan, leading to the resignation of Dr. Abebe. The new minister of health was Dr. Adenike Grange, a pediatrician who fully supported primary health care in Nigeria (interview, Samaru, 7 August 2007); but her tenure was also short-lived, as she resigned in March 2008 after charges of financial irregularities in the ministry (Abdulmalik 2008). This disruption in leadership in the Ministry of Health in 2008—at one point it was directed by the head of the Ministry of Labour—ended with the appointment of a permanent minister of health, Professor Babatunde Osotimehin, in November 2008. One month earlier, in October 2008, Mrs. Koleoso-Adelekan, a political appointee of President Obasanjo, had been dismissed and replaced by Dr. Muhammed Ali Pate, an experienced health official who had worked with the World Bank (Sam and Falola 2008).

While these discontinuities in institutional leadership may not have been apparent to parents in Zaria, they would have noticed their effects on National Immunization Day practices. After 2007, bednet distributions were abandoned, ostensibly because of a lack of funds. The USAID-funded COMPASS program, which emphasized community health dialogue and local involvement in health campaigns, ended in 2009 (Rabiu 2009). Furthermore, complaints that health workers are still not providing complete, house-to-house coverage (Joseph 2009a, 2009b) underscore some people's belief that the primary benefits of the Polio

Eradication Initiative have gone to immunization team workers and to federal, state, and local health officials.

*   *   *

Many people have lost faith in President Yar'Adua's promises to provide basic services to the nation as water and electricity have become increasingly scarce. One Islamic teacher at an immunization day program in Suleja, Niger State, in July 2008 put it this way:

> Since 1960 when we had our independence, there were five things that government always talk about—water, light, housing, food and health—but up till today, we are still in the same problem. Every government that comes will promise us that they will solve these problems, but none of them has been able to do anything meaningful. Our children keep dying without considering that these are the things that make them die. (Rabiu 2008b)

This skepticism about the Nigerian government's ability to provide basic services and primary health care has led many to rely on their own health practices and understandings, rather than on government pronouncements which they consider inconsistent and unreliable. While some people continue to refuse to allow their children to be vaccinated because they believe that the polio vaccine is contaminated with antifertility substances or HIV-AIDS, rumors about the safety of the oral polio vaccine are more complex than this simple explanation for people's refusal to participate suggests. These rumors and subsequent debates also raised questions about government's responsibility to meet the health needs of citizens, about what sorts of public health programs should be implemented, and about underlying ideologies associated with appropriate community health care.

Yet some people did believe that the polio vaccine was a form of anti-Islamic population control. Nonetheless, rumors do not always represent literal beliefs, but rather they may serve as vehicles for the airing of broader discontent. Rumors about oral polio vaccine enabled some people to express their disagreement with the way that the Polio Eradication Initiative had been implemented, including the decision to focus on polio alone through house-to-house campaigns and the establishment of a top-down public health initiative, about which they had no say, for what they perceived as a minor health problem. While polio vaccines were given free of charge, medicines for malaria had to be paid for, and other vaccines, when available, sometimes involved "incidental" expenses. By protesting the Polio Eradication Initiative as it was originally implemented, they were able to voice their discontent and to have at least some of their children's health needs addressed during Immunization Days in 2006 and 2007. Those without economic resources and with little education, who perceive malaria, measles, and meningitis as the biggest threats to the lives of their children, support public health initiatives which address these problems. That acceptance of polio immunization improved in 2006 after such concerns were addressed suggests that resistance to public health programs may be overcome when a congruence of aims and interests can be found (Delaney 1987). The subsequent political disorder at the ministry level in 2007 and 2008, however, has undermined these improvements and has contributed to distrust of government claims, reinforcing the belief that God is the most reliable source of protection. Yet the fact that, in Northern Nigeria, both those who have supported and those who have protested polio eradication efforts are Muslims suggests that immunization can have multiple interpretations according to Islamic precepts. These interpretations are examined in the following chapter.

4. Islam and Immunization in Northern Nigeria

Allah the Great and Almighty has created for each disease a remedy.

—Al-Jawziyya, *The Prophetic Medicine*

They are lost indeed who kill their children foolishly without knowledge, and forbid what Allah has given to them forging a lie against Allah; they have indeed gone astray, and they are not the followers of the right course.

— Qur'an 6:140

Hadith 11. Leave that which makes you doubt for that which does not make you doubt.

—An-Nawawi, *Forty Hadith*

While resistance to the Polio Eradication Initiative and to immunization more generally has often been attributed to the Islamic community in Northern Nigeria, Muslims have responded in a range of ways to immunization programs, reflecting different teachings and interpretations of Islamic texts as well as their different educational and socioeconomic backgrounds. Indeed, many Muslim parents consider both routine immunization and taking oral polio vaccine to be acceptable practices. For them, the main obstacle has been the lack of available vaccines (FBA Health Systems Analysts 2005). Others are willing to take their children to be vaccinated at local clinics and hospitals when specific diseases threaten and their fear of disease overshadows the risks they see in vaccination. However, some see immunization as unnecessary or even possibly dangerous for healthy infants and children, regardless of impending epidemics. For these parents, prayer is not only sufficient, but is the only real protection against disease, which ultimately comes from God. The phrase *kariya Allah,* usually translated as "natural immunity," has a different meaning in this context. In this case, it refers to the special protection (*kariya*) given by Allah, rather than to the response of the immune system exposed to a particular virus (or as opposed to immunity derived from a vaccine).[1] This latter view of immunity is supported by an influential text titled *The Prophetic Medicine,* which stresses that for every disease, God created a cure (B. Umar 2006). This cure may consist of prayer either alone or combined with specific medicinal substances, including Western medicine (*magani boko*). Thus Islamic scholars, and Muslims in Northern Nigeria more generally, are not categorically opposed to Western medicine. However, immunization—which requires the injection or ingestion of disease-laden substances (either killed or attenuated viruses)—may be seen as an unclean or harmful practice which threatens children's health. In trying to follow Islamic precepts not to harm one's children, parents need to assess the risks and benefits of vaccination; how to proceed is not always clear. That there are Muslims who have supported polio vaccination and those who have rejected it suggests that immunization does not have a single interpretation according to Islamic precepts, and this multiplicity of views has historical precedents in Northern Nigeria.

This chapter begins with a general overview of Islamic medicine as it has historically been practiced in Northern Nigeria, including measures taken to prevent disease, concepts of immunization, and the treatment of specific symptoms using traditional Hausa medicine, Western medicine, prayer, and the appeasement and exorcism of spirits (*rukiyya;* see O'Brien 2001). How immunization, in particular, is interpreted in Northern Nigeria reflects the specific political context in which Islam has emerged, the role that Islam and Shari'a law plays in local, regional, and national politics, and differences in Islamic practice. While interviews, mainly in Zaria, and archival documents suggest that the current resistance of some Muslim teachers to the distribution of oral polio vaccine continues earlier resistance to smallpox immunization campaigns, the Polio Eradication Initiative began at a time of considerable political tension and insecurity in Northern Nigeria (M. Last 2008), relating to national and international affairs. The complex responses to this sense that the Muslim community is under increasing threat are expressed in the resistance to some immunization interventions from outside, which are seen as detrimental, and in the acceptance of others, which are seen as proper and beneficial.

Islamic Medicine in Northern Nigeria

Magani abu Allah (medicine is a thing of God)

—Saying painted on the back of a bus, Zaria, 2007

From the fifteenth century, when Islam was gradually introduced into Northern Nigeria by traveling scholars and traders, until the reformist jihad of Sheikh Usman dan Fodio in 1804 and the establishment of the Sokoto Caliphate in what is now Northern Nigeria, Islamic medicine was practiced alongside Hausa medicine (Abdalla 1997). While a range of traditional Hausa medical practitioners—including *boka* (specialists in herbal medical treatment for various ailments), *mai magani* (collectors and sellers of herbal and other medicines), *unwanzani* (literally "barbers," those who performed circumcision and blood-letting), *mai dori* (specialists in bone setting), and *mai bori* (those who treated illness attributed to *bori* spirits)—provided medical services to the general population, Muslim scholars (*malamai*) from other parts of West Africa residing in Kano and other urban centers were called upon to treat ailing emirs and princes (Abdalla 1997, 102). Their work was based on written texts on *materia medica*—vegetable and mineral medical treatments—and on *The Prophetic Medicine,* a compilation of hadith (sayings of the Prophet) and portions of the Qur'an pertaining to illness which stresses the power of prayer to prevent and cure disease. These different medical systems operated in parallel until the reforms of the 1804 jihad, when certain aspects of Hausa medicine came to be viewed as un-Islamic and when Arabic texts associated with Islamic medicine became more respected and attracted a more broadly based following (Abdalla 1997, 102). Belief in the spiritual causes of disease persisted, but it began a gradual shift from belief in *bori* spirits, associated with Hausa medicine, to belief that Allah alone was the source of all illness and cure. A range of spirits—angels (*mala'ika*), jinn (*aljanu*), and the devil (*shaitan*), all under the control of Allah—were also part of this cosmology.[2] However, while Sheikh dan Fodio and his son Muhammad Bello focused on eliminating particular aspects of traditional Hausa religious practice which were used in treating or preventing illness, including divination, *bori* spirit worship, numerology, and astrology (M. Last 1967, 4–5), their reforms affected local understandings of disease only gradually. Indeed, the tentative acceptance of these changing concepts of spirits and causes of disease may be seen in a comment that Baba of Karo made about *bori* spirits to Mary Smith in 1950:

> All of the rulers like the *bori*—if they didn't, would their work be any good? Of course they all agree with them. So do the *malams,* secretly. The *malams* will call on the *bori* in private, in the darkness of the night. Everyone wants the spirits, kings and noblemen want them, *malams* and wives shut away in their compounds—it is with them that we work in this world, without them would our labor be of any use? The work of *malams* is one thing, the work of *bori* experts is another, each has his own kind of work and they must not be mixed up. There is the work of *malams,* of *bori,* of magicians, of witches; they are all different but at heart everyone loves the spirits. There are spirits of the bush animals, there are spirits of the bush trees, there are spirits of the rocks, there are spirits of the paths, there are spirits of men inside the town. (Smith 1954, 222; see Abdalla 1991, 44)

The tension between belief in the work of *malamai* and belief in the work of *bori* specialists is evident in cases of children who contracted paralytic polio, when a father would take the child to an Islamic scholar while an older grandmother would surreptitiously take the child to a *bori* healer. As one older woman explained, "They were trying to help me. And my father and his male family members were *malamai*—Muslim scholars. It was my grandmother who was getting medicine in secret, medicine such as traditional medicine from *bori* people. But God didn't make me stand up" (interview, Zaria City, 10 August 2005).

However, the situation described by this woman and by Baba of Karo no longer exists in towns such as Zaria. Rather, it is belief in *aljanu* (jinn), rather than in "pagan" *bori* spirits, that helps to explain illness and symptoms such as paralysis. These spirits are the province of *malamai*, particularly Islamic scholars trained in the Sufi tradition of Islam. While Sufism has itself been put into question by the more recent reformist Muslim religious group known as Izala (Jama'atu Izalat al-Bid'a wa Iqamat al-Sunna), which was established in Northern Nigeria in 1978

(M. Umar 1993, 167; plate 3), Sufi *malamai* continue to be consulted in many parts of the North. Indeed, Sufi practices have long been part of Islamic medicine in Northern Nigeria, having been referred to by Islamic scholars during the early nineteenth century. The writings of the early Sokoto Caliphate scholars still resonate with people's thinking about Islamic medicine in the twenty-first century.

Nineteenth-Century Hausa Islamic Medical Scholarship

The three earliest and most renowned Hausa Islamic scholars to write on medical issues in the Sokoto Caliphate were closely involved in the jihad that established it, as medicine was considered to be an integral part of the jihad's reforms. These men were Sheikh dan Fodio's brother, Abdullahi dan Fodio, and his son, Muhammad Bello, and an important jihad intellectual, Muhammad Tukur (Abdalla 1997, 103). Their written work continues to influence the thinking of Islamic scholars in Northern Nigeria on health. Their distinctive views of illness and cure are reflected in the different modern views of immunization held by specialists and the public alike.

Muhammad Tukur's main work, *Qira' al-Ahibba,* written in 1809, was deeply influenced by medieval Sufi writings on health. For him, prayer was the primary source of prevention and cure (Abdalla 1997, 104), a view supported by *The Prophetic Medicine.* Conversely, Abdullahi dan Fodio emphasized that maintaining the health of the body was akin to a form of prayer. In his work, *Masalih al-Insan al-Muta'alliqa bil Adyan wal 'Abdan* (An Important Consideration for Man Relating to Religion and Health), Abdullahi stressed the importance of consulting physicians who were knowledgeable about medical treatments that were in keeping with Shari'a law: in other words, that did not incorporate forbidden substances such as alcohol. These men also differed in their views on who could properly attend to the health of the Muslim community, as Abdalla (1997, 114) has noted:

> Abdullahi's stand vis-à-vis other religions and non-Muslim practitioners is clear in the *Masalih.* They have no place in the scheme of medical care he advocates. Unlike Tukur who, for example, was pleased to get some useful medical information from a non-Muslim practitioner, Abdullahi trusts none other than fellow Muslims with the health care of the community. To him, Hausa medicine must depend on Islamic medicine if the community is to benefit by it fully.

In his extensive writings on medicine, Usman dan Fodio's son, Muhammad Bello, combined aspects of the other two men's work as he wrote both on Prophetic medicine and on Islamic *materia medica,* drawing mainly on Middle Eastern sources (Abdalla 1997, 95). Bello strongly supported the use of Prophetic medicine, although he noted that it would only work if one had "a total and unquestioning belief in the infallibility of the Prophet and his medicine" (Abdalla 1997, 98). However, he did not oppose the use of Hausa traditional medicine (*magani gargarjiya*), nor did he rule out the use of materials and medical advice from the West. Indeed, in 1825, Bello persuaded the British explorer Hugh Clapperton to agree to bring a medical doctor with him when he returned to Sokoto (M. Last 1967, 8; Lockhart and Lovejoy 2005, 21).

Although his writing on *materia medica* focused on earlier Islamic texts whose authors came from the Middle East and North Africa, Muhammad Bello began a project to relate herbal and mineral remedies those texts described to locally available materials, and he made a listing of such materials in the local languages of Hausa, Fulani, and Tuareg (Abdalla 1997, 99). Although he did not complete this project, it suggests his concern with making Islamic medicine—in both its spiritual and material forms—available to the general public. "His aim and that of other jihad leaders was two-fold: to suppress non-Islamic practices in health care, and to improve the general health of fellow Muslims as a prerequisite for the realization of Allah's Will on earth" (Abdalla 1997, 102).

The Influence of Hausa Medical Scholars on Contemporary Interpretations of Islamic Medicine

These twin concerns, to reform health care according to Islamic precepts and to improve the health of Muslims in Northern Nigeria, may be seen in views of medical care held by modern Muslim scholars and healers. For example, the tradition of Muhammad Tukur, who stressed prayer above all other treatments, has continued in the work of Sufi healers such as Malam Husseini of Kano (plate 4), who uses his extensive knowledge of Islamic texts in prayers for those suffering from conditions caused by *aljanu*. As he explained,

> I'm only praying for the people, and the prayers come from the Qur'an and the prayers the Prophet Muhammed did. That is what I am doing to cure people. Even yesterday I cured one girl. I was in the mosque, they called me. After I finished praying then I went to the house. I saw the girl, I called her name, and she answered and she said she could not stand up. I prayed for her, and she stood up and she felt better. But as I said, I cannot do anything about Shan Inna. What I can do is, if a person is sick or a spirit enters a person's body, before it does harm to them I can do something. I can pray and the spirit will leave the person. And I don't see the spirit and I don't talk to them. (Interview, Kano, 23 July 2006)

He emphasizes prayer because he sees *aljanu* as the source of illness and their removal as the source of cure, a belief that some Muslim reformers see as anti-Islamic. Responding to such criticism, Malam Husseini described an incident by which he documents the legitimacy of his own perspective:

> There was one man, a *malam,* who said he didn't believe in spirits; he preached to people and was waving a book. When he finished preaching, the spirits took it and brought it to our *malam,* who is a believer in spirits [a Sufi]. And he called the *malam* and showed him the book. The *malam* said, "I don't know how you got the book, I never gave it to him and I never told anyone about it." I told the man that it was the spirits who brought it because he didn't believe in them. (Interview, Kano, 23 July 2006)

Yet some Muslim reformer-scholars who may not believe in spirits may nonetheless believe that Prophetic medicine is the best protection against disease.

One Izala *malam* teaching in an Islamiyya school in Zaria City explained this way of thinking, referring specifically to the oral polio vaccine: "Most of the Islamiyya *malamai* are still opposed; a few agree, but not many. The reason they disagree is that they still suspect [that there is] something in the vaccine. I am doing something for the children—prayers—so that they don't need the polio vaccine" (interview, Zaria, 22 August 2007). His rejection of the oral polio vaccine as contaminated and unsafe is related to Abdullahi dan Fodio's insistence that medical treatment be obtained from knowledgeable and trustworthy sources—in particular, from fellow Muslims.

While these emphases on prevention and treatment by prayer follow aspects of Tukur's work and to some extent that of Abdullahi dan Fodio, other Muslim scholars are more inclined toward the work of Sheikh Muhammad Bello, with his belief in the power of God to cure and in the use of *materia medica,* which may include traditional Hausa, Islamic, and Western medicine. As one scholar explained,

> Let me start by saying that Islam is not against medicine and technological development; it actually supports it. Islam encourages Muslims to go into this research. God challenges the Muslim, including the study of the moon, to study about themselves; God will ask people to reflect on His creation and for themselves. (Interview, Kaduna, 20 July 2006)

The view that both Western medicines and readings from the Qur'an and Hadith are appropriate was also put forward by a Muslim scholar in Zaria City:

> There are some verses in the Qur'an, if you read them, you can be cured or feel better. You can use even trees, even if not mentioned in the Qur'an, but they are allowed if they do not contain alcohol. . . . Any Western medicine that does not have alcohol is allowed. . . . You see I don't go to a *boka,* but if I am sick I can take tablets.

However, this man noted that immunization differed from curative medicine. He suggested that Muslim use of vaccines is neither allowed nor forbidden in all cases, but rather is conditional:

> All you are going to give, it must come from God, not from the wish of someone. It must come from God. For example, like polio [vaccine]: is it allowed in Islam or is it not allowed? As I told you, we don't have anything that talks about immunization in Islam and we can only beg God that if it [polio] exists, it should not be much. [But] you know there is something, you must do it because of the condition, even if that something is forbidden. But even that thing [that] is forbidden in Islam, you will have to do it—if it will cause much harm. . . . Anything that is forbidden, as I said, it can be done if the condition warrants. (Interview, Zaria City, 1 August 2006)

In other words, parents are justified in vaccinating their children against diseases which threaten harm.

Yet the ambiguous nature of vaccines, which are neither entirely allowed nor forbidden, has led other Islamic scholars to question their use.

Immunization does not belong in Islam because Allah has given humans in their appropriate, best form. We have been created in the best of forms, in the best of constitutions, which is seen in the mental, spiritual, and physical composition of man. They are made of many systems, including the immune system. Nature is so kind, it has endowed man with so many things. From the medical point of view, if you take medicine that isn't necessary it may disturb the chemical composition of your body.[3]

At the same time, this scholar noted that there are different opinions on the safety of vaccines. Some vaccines have proven over time to be effective, while the safety of others is questioned:

If you take something internally that is poisonous, it is sinful. But if something has been tested over the years and it has been effective, there is no prohibition. Traditional Hausa medicine is OK, provided the content is permissible. There could be different opinions, you cannot categorically say. Opinions are mainly by analogy; for instance the Qur'an says we have created man in the best of forms.[4] If this is true, then [as] someone who believes in the word of God, as stated in the Qur'an, don't put yourself in harm's way. There are some scientific studies that cast doubt on the safety of vaccines. (Interview, Kaduna, 20 July 2006)

This man's doubt about the safety of vaccines reflects new concerns about the consequences of vaccinating small children, based on his knowledge of contentions in the West that vaccines have caused autism (Colgrove 2006; Harris 2007a, 2007b; B. Umar 2006).[5] Like some parents of autistic children in the U.S., some Hausa parents question the safety of vaccines, which they see as introducing a hazardous substance into infant bodies. When asked to compare people's cooperation with the smallpox eradication campaign in the late 1960s to their resistance to the Polio Eradication Initiative, this man responded, "We are wiser now." What he meant is that people have become aware of debates in the West over the risks and benefits of vaccines. "Different opinions" about the safety of the oral polio vaccine also appear to have influenced some people's interpretations of routine immunization for other diseases, especially immunization using needles (*allura*).

Immunization and the Meaning of *Allura*

The Hausa term for immunization, *allura rigakafi,* means "needle of prevention," but it refers to vaccines administered both orally and by injection.[6] The word *allura* is also used to refer to all injected medicines intended to bring about a cure—*magani allura*—as opposed to *magani ruwa* (liquid medicines) or *kwayoyi* (tablets), which are taken orally. The term *allura rigakafi* thus distinguishes injectible and oral vaccines from *magani allura*, injections for cure. This association of vaccination with needles and injections has had ramifications.[7] While injections have been a preferred form of treatment, poorly administered or inappropriately given injections may cause infections or extensive pain and paralysis (FBA Health Systems Analysts 2005, 16; Wall 1988, 280–81; Wyatt 1984, 1992). The assessment of the term *allura* thus depends on circumstances and individual predispositions. In spite of these dangers, many people continue to insist that injections are the most efficacious treatment for certain conditions (see also Samuelsen 2001). One Zaria City woman expressed a common assessment of *allura* as medicine when she noted, "When children are given injections and they have a fever and rashes on their bodies, they will be cured immediately" (interview, Zaria City, 29 June 2007).

However, people seem to be reconsidering the efficacy and safety of injections, particularly when they are used for immunization. This reconsideration is expressed in terms of the risk of paralysis. For example, during a National Immunization Day exercise in Zamfara State in January 2007, parents agreed to let their children receive drops of polio vaccine but refused to allow them to be given hepatitis B injections on the grounds that they would cause paralysis (Olayinka 2007a). Similarly, in July 2006 I spoke with a well-known traditional healer (*boka*) working in the village of Solanke, just north of Zaria, who said that it was not spirits but rather the injections given by Western-trained medical doctors which caused paralysis. While this man seemed to oppose Western medicine (*magani boko*) generally, for professional reasons, his statement implies that some people have experienced paralysis after having received injections. Finally, in a television spot that was developed to promote the eradication of polio in Nigeria, the narrator, who was affected by paralytic polio, goes to his mother to ask what happened and how they treated the disease:

> She said, "You had fever and you were taken to the hospital for an injection. You had an injection and the next day your legs turned limp. . . . Some others thought that the injection affected your nerves. . . . We went to the hospital in Kaduna, Jos." (Sule n.d.)

The narrator goes on to interview Mohammad Sanusi Zakariya, a researcher in the Faculty of Medicine at Bayero University in Kano, as well as traditional healers in Ningi, Bauchi State, about the causes and treatment of polio paralysis. The connection his mother made between being "taken to the hospital for an injection" and the subsequent paralysis of his legs may reinforce local thinking about this relationship and about hospital worker malpractice (see also Nwuga and Odunowo 1978). These and other examples suggest that the belief that injections and paralysis are connected may be fairly widespread. The belief may derive from the experiences of those who have been paralyzed and of the healers who have treated them. Indeed, research shows that administering injections to young children during the early stages of a poliovirus infection may increase the likelihood of paralysis (Hull 2004, 696; Mansoor et al. 2005; Wyatt 1984, 1992).

Some people attributed the fear of injections and their association with paralysis to poorly trained health workers who did not know how to properly administer injections. If the injection site or the syringe is not sterile, or if a vein or nerve is damaged by the needle, infections (including boils or abscesses), nerve damage, and temporary paralysis can result (Fry 1965; Wall 1988). According to one pediatrician, people often preferred to go to chemists and private clinics to receive treatment, such as injections of chloroquine or Fansidar for malaria. One traditional bone-setter (*mai dori*) in Likoro, a village northeast of Zaria, said that he had treated cases of paralysis caused by injections. According to this man, when an injection was improperly administered, the needle severed a vein, which the bone-setter could cause to grow back with medicine (interview, Likoro, 29 July 2007). This explanation parallels the Western one that temporary paralysis is caused by an injection which damages a nerve. However, even trained medical staff may give injections incorrectly, as in the case of the young boy whose leg was temporarily paralyzed (possibly as a result of some sort of nerve damage) with which I began this book. After finding no fractures on an X-ray, a staff member at the teaching hospital gave the boy an injection in his paralyzed leg, a procedure advised against by medical textbooks (Hull 2004, 696; see also Mansoor et al. 2005).

It is thus not surprising that, hearing of others' unfortunate experiences, some parents would be wary of letting their children receive injections for immunization and even for medical treatment. Yet many Hausa people use Western medicines, including injections, and not all traditional healers are opposed to them. Rather, they see them as suitable for certain conditions, while not appropriate for others. According to Malam Husseini in Kano, *allura* are useful as medicine and do not violate Islamic precepts. However, according to him injections are ineffectual for illnesses and paralysis having to do with spiritual disorders: those caused by a spirit (*aljanu*) affecting a person because of some transgression or other reason, by someone commissioning a *boka* to send a spirit to harm someone, or by witchcraft in general. As he put it, the reasons for the connection between *allura* and paralysis were "beyond my knowledge." Yet he believed that paralysis was caused by spirits and that getting an injection in such a state was not only inefficacious but also dangerous (interview, 28 July 2007, Kano). The logic of this cultural belief may be seen the case of a woman who was paralyzed after experiencing a stroke (*shan yewar jiki*) in June 2007.

Injections, Spirits, and Paralysis

The woman had been visiting relatives in Anchau, a village east of Zaria, when she fainted and fell down. When she revived, her right side was completely paralyzed. Family members brought her back to her house in Zaria City and her husband consulted a *boka* from Ikara (another village outside of Zaria) for treatment. The healer told her not to use *magani boko* and under no circumstances to get an injection. He treated her to bring down her *hawan jini* (high blood pressure) using prayer and *rubutu*, the practice of writing portions of the Qur'an on a writing board, then washing off the ink with water that is then drunk by the patient (Soares 2005; Wall 1988); later, she remained in her room and women burned incense to keep spirits away from her. According to this way of thinking, it was high blood pressure which had caused the stroke, but it was a spirit which had caused the paralysis. While the woman's husband eventually agreed to her being treated by an Ahmadu Bello University cardiologist, he insisted that no injections be given. For as the Kano healer Malam Husseini had explained, "If an *aljanu* 'touches' a person, it is not good for a person to get an injection, because it increases the disease. . . . the spirits do not like injections" (interview, 28 July 2007, Kano).[8]

Allura (injections) have become a symbol of both the efficacy and the dangers of Western biomedicine. Indeed, if injections are poorly administered, injection sites may become infected or limbs may be temporarily paralyzed. These side effects have reinforced some parents' doubts about the benefits of certain types of Western medicine and of *allura rigakafi* in particular.

Resistance to Immunization (*Allura Rigakafi*)

Vaccination was commenced in Zaria Town with 200 children. It was not popular.

—*Gazetteer of Zaria Province*, 1919

Even before the implementation of the Polio Eradication Initiative, immunization campaigns had been resisted in Zaria and in neighboring local government areas. During the colonial period, forms of resistance such as running away reflected fear of European doctors and resentment of colonial rule, with its unequal relations of power.[9] In a more recent example, this fear was expressed in terms of "family planning." One Ahmadu Bello University pediatrician described the response of some villagers to the Expanded Programme on Immunisation in the early 1990s:

> Distrust of antifertility medicine in vaccines was much much earlier. Before 1996, there was resistance to these drugs. For example, in 1991–92 we went to one village in Zaria and we were stoned while we were attempting to do routine immunization. They said, "You are bringing infertility to our women." All in all, from the early 1990s, there was this resistance to immunization. I talked to the Emir of Zaria and Abubakar Gumi. I pleaded with him [Gumi] that he should say it in the radio broadcast—and he did say it—that the vaccine is safe, that his grandchildren have taken it.[10] It is out of respect or some kind of diplomacy, they will say, "It's ok." They will tell people but then they won't do anything. But even then, people did not accept it. (Interview, Zaria, 4 August 2006)

This distrust of routine immunization, which includes belief that vaccines are adulterated with contraceptive substances, fear that government and health care personnel may use outdated vaccines or misadminister them, and concern that vaccines may be altogether unavailable, along with misunderstanding about the number of doses needed, helps to explain the extremely low levels of immunization in Zaria City.[11] These low levels have been documented in several studies conducted by students in the Ahmadu Bello University Department of Community Medicine (Attah 2003; Bako 1978; Daiyabu 1977–78; Ekpo 1975–76). For example, in January 2002, Attah (2003, 49) found that of 339 children under five years old living in the Zaria Local Government Area, only 15 percent had had a full course of four doses of oral polio vaccine, although 59 percent had had three doses. Seven percent of children had had no doses at all.[12] Attah also collected data from the Kaduna State Ministry of Health on routine immunizations in all local government areas, including Zaria, and in no case was coverage higher than 50 percent, except for Bacillus Calmette-Guérin vaccine for tuberculosis. Routine immunization coverage in Kaduna State in 2007 was similarly low, and in the first half of that year Zaria Local Government had the lowest level of oral polio vaccine coverage (14 percent) in the entire state (WHO Kaduna 2007a).[13] One doctor attributed these low levels to a backlash against the focus on polio immunization during the Polio Eradication Initiative. But this view was countered by one Zaria City resident:

> Anyone that says Zaria residents reject immunisation is only saying something that is far from the truth. What we rejected was the Polio immunisation because we saw no reason why they were disturbing us with Polio Immunisation when they did not effectively handle killer diseases like measles. Our point of contention is that, it is only on rare occasions that one comes across death caused by Polio or even a victim of it, then why the prominence? This is what we reject, not immunisation generally. (Sa'idu and Ibrahim 2007)

This man was interviewed during the measles outbreak in Zaria City in November–December 2007. However, precisely what happened during the 2007 measles outbreak and whether it reflected resistance to routine immunization is not altogether clear.

The 2007 Measles Outbreak in Zaria City

The outbreak of measles (*bakon dauro, kyanda*) which occurred in November–December 2007 illustrates the various perspectives on immunization and responsibility for primary health care in Zaria, as well as the lack of disease surveillance there. The exact extent of the outbreak—precisely how many children contracted the disease, their immunization histories, and how many died—is unknown and was a point of contention in the press. When the outbreak was first reported in the *Daily Trust* on 5 December 2007 (Aodu 2007c), it was stated that fifty children had died. However, in an interview aired on the *Voice of America* on the same day, one state health official initially announced that there were "just one or two" deaths:

> Dr. Hamid Abdulkadir, the number two man at the Kaduna state ministry of health, under whose jurisdiction Zaria falls, says the victims were mostly children who declined recent mass vaccination campaigns. "Just a few cases of measles, about six cases, just one or two deaths, in families who have been rejecting the routine vaccinations during the polio-plus days," he noted. "This is a clear evidence that if you do not take the vaccination, you are very liable. We just need to step up our public awareness, particularly for those who are still rejecting." (da Costa 2007)

While Kaduna State and Zaria Local Government health officials sought to downplay the number of children who had died, they hastened to provide vaccines and treatments for "symptoms of the disease, which he [the Zaria Local Government Area Health Coordinator] said, appeared like measles," since "there was no laboratory test or medical confirmation that the disease was measles" (*Daily Trust* 2007).[14] From their perspective, the problem arose because parents had failed to get their children immunized during Immunization Plus Days, of which there had been seven in 2007.

Parents, in their turn, accused the government of not addressing the problem in a timely manner and of attempting to cover up the extent of the outbreak. Several newspaper accounts reported parents lining up with their children at local health clinics for measles vaccinations and treatment as they became available. One woman explained, "They used to feel better when they have had an injection because it brings out the measles that are inside the stomach. Those who like their children to have injection are more than those who don't want it" (interview, Zaria City, March 2008). Yet other parents did not bring their sick children to local hospitals or clinics, not because they distrusted medical treatment but because they feared the consequences of injections, as one Zaria City man observed:

> What the government authorities don't know is that ninety-six percent of the children killed by the disease were not taken to hospital. Some of our people believe that injection deteriorates the condition of a child suffering from measles. This is why most of the children infected were not taken to hospitals. They remain at home, either calling on traditional healers or buying orthodox medicines from chemist shops.[15] Despite the fact that I went to the hospital I still lost three children. (Sa'idu and Ibrahim 2007)

Unfortunately, some who did bring their children to hospitals or clinics did so too late to help them (Aodu 2007c). However, by mid-December, measles vaccines and treatment had been made available in sufficient quantities that the outbreak was contained.

During the outbreak, the question of who was to blame arose. Government health officials claimed that children would not have died if they had been immunized against measles. Parents countered that the government did not respond with treatment when the outbreak occurred. However, while it is likely that many of the children who died had not received measles vaccinations, it is unclear why they had not. Some parents may have wanted to immunize their children but could not obtain either the vaccine or transportation to vaccination sites (FBA Health Systems Analysts 2005). Others did not know what vaccines their children had received (interview, Zaria City, March 2008). It is also possible that some children had been immunized but nonetheless contracted the disease (Aaby 1995), as was explained by one Zaria City woman in 2005:

> Yes, I did take my children for immunization—I even took one of my daughters until she was five years old. But at last I stopped taking them. For example, the measles immunization. I took my children, but they had measles and it was very dangerous, more than those who hadn't gotten immunized. Really, it changed my thinking. That was why I stopped taking the other children; the immunization had no use. (Interview, Zaria City, August 2005)[16]

Health officials responded to the 2007 measles outbreak by insisting that parents needed to immunize their children, but they did so without taking parents' experiences of these vaccines and their concerns about their safety into account. Yet as Nichter has maintained (1995, 625),

> Assumptions that mothers who are non-acceptors of vaccinations (or identified as "vaccination drop-outs") have lower levels of concern about their children's health has been questioned. To the contrary, I have argued that it is often health concerns which lead child caretakers to selectively use or turn down vaccination services available to them.

Parents' distrust of government health officials was exacerbated not only by their attempts to downplay the problem but also by their failure to take parents' perspectives and experiences of immunization seriously. One official was quoted as blaming parents for not getting their children immunized because they were "attaching religious sentiments to it"; in other words, Muslim parents were not allowing immunization teams into their homes (Babadoko 2007b). While this official later denied making this statement (Sa'idu and Ibrahim 2007), his remark and denial underscore the complexity of social interactions between Muslim parents and health officials in the North.

Politics and Islamic Interpretations of Immunization

Despite this health official's claim that Muslim parents in Northern Nigeria refuse to vaccinate their children, many prominent Muslim political, religious, and educational leaders in Northern Nigeria, including the Emir of Zaria, Alhaji Shehu Idris; the Emir of Kano, Alhaji Ado Bayero; the late Sultan of Sokoto, Muhammadu Maccido; Umaru Shehu (the former WHO director for East and Southern Africa and emeritus professor of community medicine at the University of Maiduguri); the current president of Nigeria, Umaru Yar'Adua; and the former minister of health and Senate majority leader, Dr. Dalhatu Tafida (Okpani 2003a), have all supported childhood immunization and have promoted the implementation of the Polio Eradication Initiative in various ways. Both the Emir of Zaria and the Emir of Kano have participated in National Immunization Days, while the late Sultan of Sokoto issued a statement confirming the safety of the oral polio vaccine (*Daily Trust* 2004b). President Yar'Adua fully supports Immunization Plus Days, and as governor of Katsina State he occasionally accompanied teams providing polio immunization in the state. In July 2007, the secretary general of Jama'atu Nasril Islam, the umbrella organization for Muslims in Nigeria, announced that it fully supported polio eradication efforts in Nigeria (Aodu 2007b). Furthermore, the president of the International Fiqh Council, Sheikh Yusuf al-Qaradawi, disapproved of Kano Islamic leaders who had opposed the Polio Eradication Initiative, saying that "the lawfulness of such vaccine in the point of view of Islam is as clear as sunlight" and that the members of the Supreme Council of Shari'a Nigeria who opposed it were distorting "the image of Islam" (Jegede 2007).

Professor Shehu, who was the first chairman of the National Programme on Immunization and who has vigorously supported the Polio Eradication Initiative, participated in tests that confirmed the safety of the oral polio vaccine in South Africa during the 2003–2004 Kano State boycott of the Initiative. In an interview published in the *Daily Trust* in 2007, Professor Umaru noted that

> in any reasonable society, when such questions arise (on safety of OPV), you look for the people who are knowledgeable and best placed to give an opinion.... For one reason or the other, people tend to look beyond Nigeria (for expert opinion). One of the initial problems we had was that people were looking to the internet where they download archaic information; that people contract other diseases when they were immunized. (Bego 2007)

In his view, this use of material from the Internet was irresponsible and often self-interested. He also made light of claims that the West was using the polio vaccine to reduce the fertility of Muslim populations: "If America wants to do that, they will use polio to fight the Muslim World? They are still fighting the Muslim World. Polio or no polio, they have the atomic bomb." In his opinion, "there is no excuse for any child to be paralyzed as a result of polio in Nigeria today" (Bego 2007).

These men's support for childhood immunization and the Polio Eradication Initiative reflects their sincere belief in the safety of these vaccines, which, in the face of endemic wild poliovirus and epidemics of measles in Northern Nigeria, they see as critical to saving children's lives and promoting their well-being. Yet even their advice may be ignored, in part because people living in poor housing, without adequate sanitation or clean water, with low-paying jobs, and with malnourished children do not find them credible.[17] While immunization may be important for "big people" (*manya manya*) and may strengthen their credibility with Western donors, it is irrelevant to ordinary people (*talakawa*) in their day-to-day efforts to provide sufficient food, clothing, medication, and housing to their families. Furthermore, the ideals of pious religious leaders such as Sheikh dan Fodio, who "throughout his life had lived simply, with only a few clothes and with plain food and accommodation" (M. Last 1967, 9), contrast starkly with the luxurious residences, fleets of Mercedes Benzes, and frequent overseas travel of some present-day religious and political leaders. The contrast fosters both resentment of those who have access to the pleasures of Western modernity and rejection of their advice and lifestyles. Even those who have accepted immunization, including that provided through the Polio Eradication Initiative, may be displeased with the increasing disparities in wealth and well-being and come to question the religious values of their leaders. As one man from a village outside of Zaria explained, "People think government and even Muslim scholars, they have no fear of God in their minds.... Both the *malamai* and the big people now, they are not honest. They spoiled the world" (interview, Yakasai, 3 August 2006).[18] By following Muslim precepts as they have been outlined by Sheikh Usman dan Fodio and his son, Muhammad Bello (and some would add more recent reformers, such as Sheikh Abubakar Gumi [M. Umar 1993]), they hope to rebuild their sense of a moral community, in which concern for the health of the Muslim *ummah* (community) is fundamental.

Religion, Health, and International Politics

This rebuilding of community often entails a rejection of Western ways and, at times, an intolerance of other points of view, as one Ahmadu Bello University physician observed:

> The political [situation] has become much more cloudy. Before, people were more tolerant; one could discuss these issues in a public forum. As it is now, because of this animosity, if a Muslim is saying something against a *malam,* he is not a good Muslim. Or if a Christian says something, it is not to be accepted. (Interview, Zaria, 4 August 2006)

However, this rejection is also fueled by outside events and the fears that they have engendered. The conjunction of the implementation of national population policies in the late 1980s with pressures to implement the Expanded Programme on Immunisation in Nigeria have led some to question the sincerity of Western-supported health programs. As one Ahmadu Bello University Islamic legal scholar explained,

> You know, about forty years back, America, Britain, and other European nations were respected. Because I, too, I remember when I was a boy, I used to hear about President Kennedy every day on the radio, and this President Kennedy, he was acceptable among our people. After Kennedy, when he was shot, people were very, very sad—they were grieved. . . . But towards this Iranian Revolution and from what we hear from Iran, we hear from Iran all over the world, pamphlets were circulating asking Muslims to be alert, that America and Britain were all out to destroy Muslims. Going through some of these pamphlets . . . there was declassified information that actually stated that the Muslim population was growing, the American population was diminishing. They targeted the youth deficit because [American] women were no longer interested in producing children. According to some highlights in the security memorandum,[19] if this was allowed to go unchecked, America and other nations would be overrun by the Muslim countries. . . . So the best way [to address this problem] is to check the population. (Interview, Zaria, 30 July 2006)

This distrust of the motives of the West is supported by a range of publicly available materials—international newspaper and journal articles, radio broadcasts, and pages on the World Wide Web—and has been reinforced by the continuing American presence in the Middle East. As this man noted, "Because [of this presence], most of the places I attend, Muslims are always against the war—this had made them against anything coming from the U.S." This rejection of "anything coming from the U.S." has carried over into questioning the safety of Western biomedicine in general (M. Last 2005, 561). Traditional Hausa or Islamic medicine provides what many consider a safer health option. While distrust of biomedicine was not the primary impetus for the establishment of a Muslim Specialist Hospital in Zaria in 1999—it was founded to address the problems of mistreatment or neglect of Muslim patients by Christian physicians—only Muslim doctors provide biomedical treatment there.

Another consequence of Muslim distrust of Western-sponsored medical interventions and of those associated with such interventions (the *'yan boko* described by a local community leader in the previous chapter) has been suspicion of immunization—often expressed in terms of fears of injections—and of the Polio Eradication Initiative. According to one Muslim scholar, Hadith 11, "Leave that which makes you doubt for that which does not make you doubt," means that the *malamai* teaching married women and children in Islamiyya schools have a duty "to protect their subjects" by advising them to refuse vaccination (interview, Kaduna, 20 July 2006).

*　*　*

There is not a monolithic Islamic view on immunization within Northern Nigeria.[20] Rather, depending on their education and social class, as well as particular readings and understandings of the Qur'an and the Hadith, parents have or have not had their children immunized against polio and other childhood diseases. Furthermore, the distinctive histories of those living in Northern Nigeria and cultural interpretations of different forms of medical practice—Hausa, Islamic, and Western—have influenced Muslim men and women's views of the politics of immunization and international conflict, of government responsibility for primary health care—including the provision of basic services such as clean water and sanitation—and of inequalities in wealth, education, and living standards.

One striking aspect of Northern Nigerian Muslims' varied views on immunization is the enduring influence of the writings of the early nineteenth-century jihad scholars. For example, Muhammad Bello's vision of medicine as providing for the well-being of the entire Muslim community is echoed in the comments of the elderly man who decried the greed of the politicians and Islamic scholars who have "spoiled the world" by only thinking of themselves. Also, the importance of prayer (discussed by Muhammad Tukur and Muhammad Bello) and the influence of spirits (described by Sheikh Usman dan Fodio and Muhammad Bello) are reflected in the thinking of Sufi *malamai* and Hausa traditional healers, whose amulets include portions of the Qur'an and may be used to protect against malicious spirits (Wall 1988; see also Marty 1914). Furthermore, Abdullahi dan Fodio's insistence that Muslims' health is best attended to by fellow Muslims may be seen in the establishment of the Muslim Specialist Hospital and in the preference for vaccines made in Islamic countries. Alternatively, Muhammad Bello's acceptance of Western sources of medical knowledge and practice is evident in the remarks of Professor Shehu on the value of vaccines, although his comment that one should "look for the people who are knowledgeable and best placed to give an opinion" about a disease and its cure parallels the words of Abdullahi dan Fodio written a century earlier. In Northern Nigeria, a long religious history underlies these different views and concerns.

One group of Muslims who share Muhammad Bello's pragmatism about Western medicine and who fully support the Polio Eradication Initiative and routine immunization in Northern Nigeria are those who have been disabled by polio themselves. Because of their own experience of polio, they see these practices as good for the Muslim community, even while others distrust them. One recent change in the Initiative has been the incorporation of people with polio in the campaign during Immunization Plus Days events, although this change was not continued. However, the Nigerian government and NGOs such as USAID are supporting efforts by people disabled by polio—the lame, *guragu*—to obtain Western education, which many Northern Nigerians, regardless of their different views on Western biomedicine, see as beneficial. By offering Western education (*ilimi boko*) along with Islamic education (*allo* and Islamiyya) to those disabled by polio, organizations such as the Polio Victims Trust Association hope to provide alternative occupations to begging for alms. These efforts are examined in the next chapter.

5. Polio, Disability, and Begging

Did He not find you poor and enrich you?
So do not oppress the orphan, and do not drive the beggar away,
And keep recounting the favours of your Lord.

—Qur'an 92:8–11

In the attempt to find work for thousands of unemployed who were healthy and normal, it is not surprising that little was done for the rehabilitation of the handicapped.

—Schram, *A History of the Nigerian Health Services*

You are normal only if you are well-educated.

—Sarkin Guragu Zazzau

Like concepts of disease and medicine, the perception and treatment of those who have been paralyzed by polio in Northern Nigeria reflects Islamic ideals and practices. Indeed, what it means to be disabled, as well as what it means to be "normal" (in the sociological sense used by Goffman [1963, 5]), reflects the larger social and cultural context of a community. In Nigeria, how a physical disability such as lameness is experienced is greatly influenced by ethnicity. In Yoruba society, lame family members were until recently kept at home for fear of the family's reputation being spoiled, while in Hausa society, disability was seen as something from God and was not, in and of itself, socially stigmatizing.[1] This view of disability has other implications as well. For just as disability is something from God, so is good fortune, so that individuals are encouraged to share their wealth—to give alms (*sadaka*) to the poor and to those whose physical condition makes it difficult to work. Indeed, charitable alms-giving, both the informal *sadaka* and the institutionalized *zakkat* (alms given during Ramadan), is one of the five primary obligations of Islam (Wall 1988, 101–103). A consequence of this principle is that until recently, most parents of children paralyzed by polio expected that their male children would earn their livelihood as beggars. This social dynamic is clarified by an examination of the ways that the lame (*guragu*), whose disability is often a result of polio (Daniel 1978), have been imagined and treated within the larger Hausa context of alms-giving and begging. Men and women who contracted polio during the early 1930s had different experiences, reflecting local gender mores. For boys, growing up lame at that time often meant learning how to beg and traveling in Nigeria and beyond as part of the Hausa trade network, which was facilitated by the building of the colonial railroad and road system. For girls, it meant staying at home until marriage brought them to their husbands' houses, as the social mores of seclusion discouraged married women from appearing in public to beg. While colonial government officials in Ghana within the Department of Social Welfare and Community Development were concerned with begging and generated an official report (Anonymous 1955), little was done in Ghana or in Nigeria, either during the colonial era or soon after Independence, to train the physically handicapped for other types of work (Rehabilitation of beggars, Nigerian National Archives).

However, in the 1980s changing perceptions of begging and alms-giving and new opportunities for the lame, especially education, led the parents of some polio-disabled children to place them in schools. The possibility of getting an education and subsequently a job—of leading a "normal life" (*zaman daidai*)— muted the possibility that stigma (*abin kunya;* literally, "something shameful") would be associated with lameness and begging. In recent years, these educated individuals themselves have sought to fund the schooling of more disabled children, to form new organizations which advocate disability rights, and to promote business schemes for the polio-disabled which would allow them to earn enough money to stop begging. These changes, as well as the social welfare programs supported by the federal government and NGOs which make these changes possible, are then considered. By seeking education and regular forms of work, the polio-disabled have been able to avoid the social stigma which is associated with begging but not with lameness itself.

Programs specifically for the polio-disabled have been expanded to include vocational training and microcredit loans. Polio-disabled people also participated for a time in the Polio Eradication Initiative, when programs such as the USAID-sponsored Community Participation for Action in the Social Sector (COMPASS) shifted their strategy to include more community input in the campaign, setting up and registering organizations such as the Polio Victims Trust Association with state governments. While the COMPASS program provided resources for polio victims, it also made those who had been affected by paralytic polio more visible to parents who refused to vaccinate their children, undermining some parents' claims that polio was not a threat to their community (Veenman and Jansman 1980, 39). Several polio-disabled people felt strongly that those who had experienced polio firsthand were in a better position to convince parents to immunize their children and were pleased when the COMPASS program personnel approached them in 2006 about working with immunization teams. Although expenses and logistical difficulties had reduced their inclusion in the Immunization Plus Day exercises by the next year, they remain strong supporters of the Polio Eradication Initiative. They also remain involved with other projects supported by the federal government and the Kano and Kaduna State governments.

Being *Gurgu* or *Gurguwa*

The word *gurgu* or *gurguwa*, "lame" (the masculine and feminine forms; the plural is *guragu*), refers to all people with physical handicaps associated with paralysis or amputation of a limb or limbs. Those with other disabilities, such as blindness (*makafi*) or disfigurement caused by leprosy (*kutare*), have their own organizations (Cohen 1969, 44–45) and have been treated differently from *guragu* by government and NGO programs (Rehabilitation of beggars, Nigerian National Archives). While not all people classified as *guragu* became lame as a result of polio, many who became paralyzed when they were very young are likely to have had polio.

Views of the lame in Hausa proverbs and songs suggest that in the past, the lame were not viewed sympathetically. Proverbs such as *Gurgu ba ya koyawa gurgu tafiya* ("The lame will not teach the lame to walk"; Whitting 1940, 61) and *Gurgu shina gani a kan sari sanda a duka shi da ita* ("The lame man has to look on while the stick is cut with which he is beaten"; Johnston 1966, 104), while they admonish listeners not to offer advice without knowledge and not to put themselves in harm's way, also suggest that the lame were viewed as helpless victims, who could only "look on" and not actively improve themselves. This view may be related to the belief that paralysis was caused by possession by the *bori* spirit Shan Inna, who left victims' limbs shriveled and useless (see chapter 3), or by the machinations of those with witchcraft medicines (*sammu*), which could cause a range of afflictions (Wall 1988, 140). While *bori* spirits might be appeased or evil intentions countered, once paralysis had continued for some time it was considered irreparable.

This view of lameness changed somewhat with the shift away from belief in *bori* spirits and toward more exclusively Islamic practice. The Qur'an enjoins people to show sympathy for the disabled, including the lame: "There is no harm if the blind, the lame, the sick, or you yourselves, eat in your own houses or the houses of your fathers, mothers, or your brothers' houses" (24:61). By treating the disabled as part of one's family, one acknowledges a common humanity in misfortune—all human beings are subject to the will of Allah, and people with disabilities are not victims of blood-drinking spirits or of the perpetrators of witchcraft. Becoming lame has come to be viewed as one's allotment in this world, just as being wealthy or having a special skill is the result of Allah's will. Furthermore, this way of viewing the lame does not rule out their self-improvement or education, as several Islamic scholars mentioned (interview, Kaduna, 20 July 2006).

However, this view of good fortune and affliction implies a particular way of addressing these disparities, namely by giving alms to those who are less well off. The social dynamic of alms-giving and begging has been a primary feature of Hausa society throughout Nigeria and West Africa. For example, Abner Cohen (1969, 42), in his study of the Hausa community in the southwestern Nigerian city of Ibadan in the 1960s, noted, "By far the most institutionalized arrangement for social security in the [Hausa] Quarter is that of begging," while Wall (1988, 103) observed in the 1980s that "charitable offerings and personal intervention form virtually the only social services in Hausaland." For those who have been blessed with good fortune, distributing alms provides a way of observing the Qur'anic injunction to be generous and to alleviate suffering, giving thanks by assisting others, according to sura 30:39: "What you give on interest to increase (your capital) through others' wealth, does not find increase with God; yet what you give (in alms and charity) with a pure heart, seeking the way of God, will be doubled." Begging for alms allows the lame to maintain themselves and their families. Indeed, begging may provide more income than other types of work (Fassin 1991, 269). This fact distressed colonial officials and, subsequently, Nigerian administrators who sought to prevent begging, seeing it as hindering modern development and civic pride:

> This problem [of begging] affects the nation, our visitors and in fact all who walk along the streets. The public conscience is quickly stirred and tends to blame the Government for failure to deal adequately with the problem. We all admit it is a national disgrace which ought to be eradicated. (Rehabilitation of beggars, Nigerian National Archives)

Consequently, both before and after Independence, attempts have been made to assess the extent of begging in Hausa communities in order to develop programs to eliminate it.

Begging and Associations of the Lame

One of the earliest surveys of Hausa beggars was actually conducted in Ghana, not in Nigeria. In July–August 1954, a study of begging and destitution was carried out in ten Ghanaian cities by the colonial Department of Social Welfare and Community Development. Of a total of 596 beggars and destitute people identified and interviewed, 353 "were Hausa people and of these 273 were classed as Professional Beggars." Indeed, the authors of the report referred to the Hausa beggars as

> what might be termed the tourist traffic from Northern Nigeria, particularly Sokoto. . . . Information supplied by the Zongo [Hausa neighborhood] Chiefs and by these beggars themselves, showed that they walked to Kano, travelled free on the train to Lagos, begging in towns en route. In Lagos they begged again until they had money to pay their fare to Accra. Occasionally they travelled free or for a reduced fare if their condition appealed to the lorry driver's sympathy. (Anonymous 1955, 4)

By "professional beggars," the report meant disabled people, mainly men, who had places to sleep, either with family or with Zongo chiefs, and whose income was comparable with that of unskilled laborers. Begging was indeed a profession for these men, and they worked in particular areas at specific times, such as in motor-parks (where buses and taxis wait to collect passengers) in the morning and near mosques on Friday afternoons.[2]

I spoke with several older polio-disabled men living in Zaria and its environs who had traveled to different parts of Nigeria in this way. One man, Alhaji Garba Hassan, had taken the same route described in the Ghanaian survey (map 5.1). His description of how he traveled and where he stayed parallels the survey. One aspect of his travels that was not mentioned in the survey, however, was his organizational work with associations of the lame, the *kungiyar guragu,* which developed during this period.

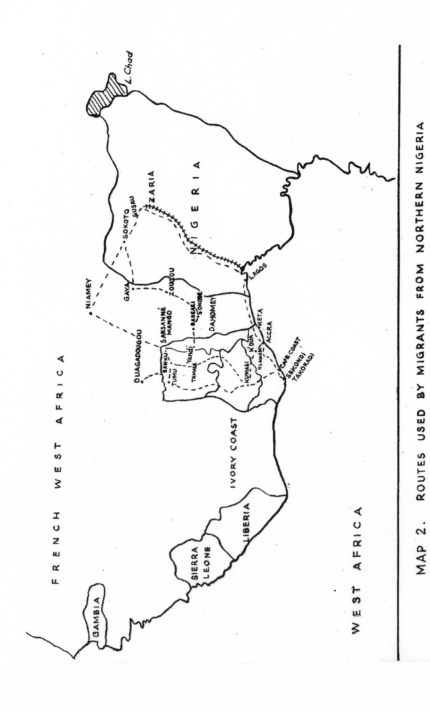

MAP 2. ROUTES USED BY MIGRANTS FROM NORTHERN NIGERIA

Map 5.1. Map of routes taken by Northern Nigerian men to Ghana in the early 1950s, from the *Report on the Enquiry into Begging and Destitution in the Gold Coast, 1954* (Anonymous 1955, iii).

Establishing Kungiyar Guragu *in Nigeria and West Africa*

Alhaji Garba (plate 5) was deeply involved in the establishment of Nigerian *kungiyar guragu* associations. According to him, the first *kungiyar guragu* group in Nigeria was founded in Lagos in 1959 by a Hausa man living in Ikare, Ekiti State, who became the first *sarkin guragu* (literally, "king of the lame"). Alhaji Garba traveled to Ikare and other southern Nigerian towns—Akure, Ilesa, Ile-Ife, Abeokuta, Agege, and Ibadan—to help establish *kungiyar guragu* groups among physically disabled Hausa living there.[3]

In the early 1960s, Alhaji Garba and the *sarkin guragu* from Ikare traveled to Kaduna in order to help establish groups in Northern Nigeria:

> It was Sarkin Ikare who turbaned the first *sarkin guragu* [in Zaria]. The Sarkin Ikare asked me to be the first *madaki guragu* [commander-in-chief], but I said no. Because I didn't want to stay in Ikare. I had my wife and children in Yakasai [near Zaria]. In 1962, *sarkin guragu* of Kano was turbaned after Ikare—followed by Ibadan, Agege, Sokoto, Katsina, and Ile-Ife. (Interview, Yakasai, 30 August 2005)

Alhaji Garba did not travel only in Nigeria. Like many Hausa migrant men who work as traders during the dry season, when they cannot farm, he went to other countries in West Africa, including Ghana and Côte d'Ivoire. Since he had been paralyzed by polio since he was seven years old, he relied on railroads and motor vehicles to get from place to place. The railroad from Lagos to Kano, which had been completed in 1912, not only brought needed primary commodities such as cotton to Lagos on the coast, where they could be shipped to England, but also enabled Northern Nigerians to travel to the south. For disabled people, this situation was particularly beneficial as they were allowed to travel free of charge.

Alhaji Garba himself traveled this route from Zaria on his way to Ghana in the early 1960s. First he went by train to Lagos, where he stayed with the *sarkin guragu* of Lagos while begging. He then went to Ghana by road:

> I went to Dahomey [at Porto Novo], then Togo, then Accra [Ghana]; from Accra I went to Kumasi, and I went to Côte d'Ivoire, that is Abidjan. I went to Bamako [Mali], and then Ouagadougou [Burkina Faso]. Then I came back to Kumasi. I went there to put the heads of our people [Hausa disabled people] together so there won't be differences. (Interview, Yakasai, 30 August 2005)

While in Côte d'Ivoire, he was trading and making shoes as well as begging. When he returned to Nigeria he first stayed in Lagos and then in 1963 moved back to Yakasai, where he built a house and married. He is no longer working because of his poor eyesight, but he remains active in the Kungiyar Guragu Zazzau, attending meetings in Zaria City every Sunday morning.

A Meeting of the Kungiyar Guragu Zazzau

The Kungiyar Guragu Zazzau was first organized in 1985 and registered with the local government in 2004. It was founded by ten men in order to help one another by raising funds to cover expenses associated with illnesses and funerals. They have subsequently met with government officials to let them know of their problems and concerns. At a meeting on Sunday, 17 July 2005, approximately forty people—most of whom were middle-aged, although there were several younger men and two small boys, as well as one very old, white-haired man—met in one of the local government offices in the center of Zaria City. All had some type of physical handicap, although they did not always know whether polio was the cause of their disabilities. During the meetings, funds were collected to help individuals during illness or with the expense of naming ceremonies and weddings. Association leaders also discussed recent applications for local, state, and federal funds for various projects for their members, including the completion of a workshop in Zaria where members are to be trained and given employment. They planned visits to other *kungiyar guragu* in Kaduna and Kano and a trip to the turbaning of the new head of the Kaduna State organization in August. Like associations based on occupation or educational background, the group has both social and financial aspects.

A topic that was not discussed at this meeting was begging. Many of the group's members worked at least part-time as beggars. Indeed, after I attended this meeting, I began to recognize association members as they sat at corners near major intersections in town. Like members of other organizations for the disabled in Zaria, such as the Kungiyar Kutare and Kungiyar Makafi, members have specific begging sites and times, which other disabled beggars respect (Ogala 1971, 6).[4] The Sarkin Guragu Zazzau explained that while many of the group's members beg, they do so because they lack training to perform other forms of work: "There are children who have polio and are not educated. But we are in democracy now; if government will help us to have education for our children, they will not suffer by doing begging. Because of poverty, they have nothing to do but beg" (interview, Zaria City, 16 July 2005). Similarly, Alhaji Garba remarked, "I don't like the idea of going for *bara* [begging]—and most of us, we don't like it. If you have something to do, you can leave it" (interview, Yakasai, 3 August 2006). For him, being disabled limits the type of work one can do, but if the disabled have training they can stop begging. Some *guragu* in Zaria who had worked as beggars have been able to amass sufficient funds, either from family or patrons, to do other sorts of work. Malam Shui'abu, for instance, now runs an Islamic school. But receiving training to practice a trade does not guarantee financial success; in such cases a reduction in the stigma of begging may be offset by an inability to earn enough to live on.

Reassessing Disability, Begging, and Stigma

Begging is being reassessed in Northern Nigeria. Once seen as condoned by Islam as a form of social support for the disabled, it is now considered shameful. This shift reflects changing ideas about the lame that are associated with increased literacy, with continuing government attempts to eliminate begging through education and vocational training, and with international attention to the disabled.

Because of the difficulty of travel in the early twentieth century, particularly for those living in small villages in Zaria Province, lameness was understood to mean vulnerability and the inability to work. Disabled men who were lame married later, because it took them longer to raise funds for the necessary parental and bridal gifts. Furthermore, as Alhaji Garba noted, "People didn't want their daughters to marry *guragu*. . . . If they are illiterate, they would think that if they marry their daughter to a *gurgu,* she can contract it." Women *gurgu* married young—around 12–14 years of age. Once married, they remained in their husbands' houses as the practice of seclusion in Zaria City requires, unless accompanied by their husbands. I interviewed two older *gurguwa* women; both were married to *gurgu* men and both had given birth to "normal" children, without disabilities.[5] However, younger men (and perhaps women) with education and financial resources can now, as Alhaji Garba noted, "marry when they like, either *guragu* or *lafiya* [the lame or the healthy]." This shift to seeing the lame as eligible marriage partners suggests a transformation in thinking about *guragu* more generally; lameness no longer nec-essarily means helplessness or stigma. Alhaji Garba observed that parents who re-fused to marry their daughters to polio-disabled men were not concerned "about shame, about stigma [*abin kunya*], it's just about illiteracy" (interview, Yakasai, 3 August 2006) and that parents who thought that way were simply uneducated.[6]

What is shameful or stigmatizing, however, is begging. For example, one older man in Zaria City, who was polio paralyzed as a child, as were his two wives, has healthy children for whom he is responsible and has supported by beg-ging. Yet he noted, "It's very embarrassing for my children and grandchildren to see me and my wives begging, so we want some sort of work so we can support ourselves" (interview, Zaria City, 16 July 2005).[7]

Since many older polio-disabled people had no Western education—indeed, their families had encouraged them to beg at an early age rather than attend school—begging was the only work they were able to do. However, not all men and women who had been paralyzed by polio when very young had been com-pelled to beg as children. I interviewed eleven physically disabled individuals in Zaria in 2005 and found that age, gender, and socioeconomic status, as well as the presence or absence of a critical individual supporting Western education for a disabled child, were important factors in determining whether the child was sent to beg. Of the four men who had never begged, all were under forty-five years of age and three had been given a Western education by their parents. One older woman had never begged because her parents (and later her husband) did not allow her to do so. All six who were then begging or had done so in the past were over fifty-five, and none had received Western education as children (al-though two men had taken adult education classes). The one woman who begged did so with her husband, who was also lame.

For those who are young and disabled but without resources, the difficulties of attending school and of securing employment are evidenced by the occasional ap-peals published in Nigerian newspapers highlighting the plight of particular indi-viduals. In one piece published in August 2007, a sixteen-year-old young man who begs in Abuja, the national capital, "said [that] if Nigerians could come to his aid, he would quit begging because it goes contrary to the doctrine of his religion (Islam)." His assessment of his condition exemplifies the way that begging is being recast as something no longer acceptable to Muslims, while the inability to walk is something that, being from Allah, should serve as a lesson to others: "People should use my situation to fear Allah, to understand that there is Allah and the last day. For the past 16 years of my life, I have been moving by rolling. That does not mean that Allah hates me, but it is his wish to create me like this" (Shuaibu 2007, 35). While not all Muslims in Northern Nigeria would agree that begging is un-Islamic, many younger disabled people and Nigerian government officials do, as evidenced in efforts to reduce or eliminate begging both in the 1960s and, in Abuja, since 2003.

Government Attempts to Reduce Begging in Northern Nigeria

Federal and state government officials have tried several times to establish rehabilitation programs in order to end the practice of begging. For example, in the 1950s, British colonial officials sought to rehabilitate disabled workers, but because responsibility for the scheme was shunted off to different agencies, little was accomplished (Employment of Disabled People, Nigerian National Archives). In 1966, members of the Nigerian Ministry of Social Welfare and Community Development, along with prominent community members (including several traditional rulers), met to discuss how best to address the problem of begging in the Northern Provinces. They considered organizing rehabilitation and training centers in Kano, Jos, and Kaduna, but did not think it would be possible to fund and staff them (Rehabilitation of beggars, Nigerian National Archives). Their report resulted in the formation of the voluntary Association for the Rehabilitation of the Disabled, headed by the Emir of Kano and with Nigerian members of the International Red Cross on its board. However, their long-term goal of setting up a residential rehabilitation and training center was never attained, in part because of the outbreak of civil war in 1967.

Three aspects of the committee's work reflected changes in opinion about begging. First, committee members (many of whom were Muslims themselves) sought to discourage the practice of giving alms directly to individual Muslims:

> With the clearing of the beggars from the streets, people may find no outlet for their pleasure in alms-giving. It is therefore recommended that some form of Trust Fund be started where willing givers can make their regular or periodical contributions. Collections from Zakkat, Churches and Mosques will be paid to this Fund. The public should be trained and encouraged to support the Fund by gifts in cash or kind. The proceeds could be used to provide additional comfort such as clothing, games, sports outfit and equipment etc. for inmates or the provision of tools for outgoing inmates to commence independent living.

Second, the they sought to decouple begging from Islam:

> We have been assured that Islamic theology and religion views begging as an authorized evil. However, according to the Moslem religion and law, Islam enjoins

everybody to work for a living and that although the giving of alms is not prohibited, it is supposed to be channeled through the state.

Third, the acting permanent secretary of the Ministry of Economic Planning, on reviewing the committee's report, noted that while funds used rehabilitating beggars might not have the overall impact of other health interventions,

> there is the fact that the rehabilitation of these beggars may raise the morale of the entire population and project the image of Nigeria favourably from the international viewpoint. (Rehabilitation of beggars, Nigerian National Archives)

Despite the committee's hopes, alms-giving has not been "channelled through the state" or centralized in a trust fund. However, the hope of the ridding the streets of beggars, whose presence is associated with backwardness and poverty, in order to improve the image of the modern Nigerian state in the international community has been a primary impetus for rehabilitating the disabled. This association of modernity with clean and orderly surroundings, in which beggars constitute a sort of "social dirt" (in the sense of people out of appropriate place), is reflected in recent efforts to rid the federal capital, Abuja, of beggars by moving them to rehabilitation villages outside of Abuja or returning them to their hometowns.

The Removal, Rehabilitation, and Return of Abuja Beggars

After Nasir Ahmad el-Rufai was appointed minister of the Federal Capital Territory in 2003, he began to implement a program to remove beggars from Abuja and send them to the Bwari School for Rehabilitating Beggars, where they would be housed, trained for jobs, and provided with amenities such as electricity and running water. The program was only temporarily successful:

> As efforts to restore the FCT's master plan and transform it into one of the neatest cities in the world went on, residents of Abuja woke up one morning to find beggars cleared off the streets of FCT to the rehabilitation school at Bwari Area Council in the Federal Capital Territory. . . . Barely three months to the end of el-Rufai's tenure, some of the achievements of the former minister are gradually becoming a thing of the past, one of which is the stylish return of beggars to the streets of Abuja. (Hassan 2007, 52)

It is perhaps appropriate that it was officials of the Abuja Environmental Protection Board, rather than of the Ministry of Social Welfare and Community Development (as in the 1960s) or the Department of Labor (as in the 1950s: Employment of Disabled People, Nigerian National Archives) who were most directly involved in this attempt to remove beggars from the streets, since the goal of this program was to transform Abuja into "one of the neatest cities in the world," rather than to help the disabled.

However, the plan has run into problems. Because the rehabilitation village was remote and there was little money for farming or other work in the area, residents who remained found it difficult to sustain themselves (J. Abubakar 2007, 37).[8] Some of those who returned to their hometowns to ply their newly learned trades could not support themselves either, as was the case for one man from Zamfara State, to the northeast:

"I was one of the beggars rehabilitated at the Bwari School for Rehabilitating Beggars established in el-Rufai's time. I was taught how to make leather shoes before I was repatriated to Zamfara which I spent almost a year until I finally returned to Abuja when this new government was sworn-in."

Explaining why he returned, Baba said, "I was not doing well in the shoe making business because of lack of capital and people were not patronising me. I spent all that I got during my stay in Abuja. I was skeptical about returning to Abuja at first for the fear of being arrested by the authority, especially when I heard that new ministers have been nominated; [it was] for the fear that el-Rufai may be retained which made me to buy a small radio set to be current."

. . . According to him, he is still grateful to the former minister for giving him the opportunity to learn a trade but he prefers begging because he makes more money as he described FCT residents as generous people. (Hassan 2007, 52)

Despite these difficulties in addressing the problem of begging, international concern with the condition of the disabled has led to new, less coercive programs for providing education and vocational training being developed in several Northern Nigerian states.

International Initiatives for Disability Rights and Programs for the Disabled in Kaduna State

Recent international initiatives, such as the UN Decade for the Disabled (1983–92), have called attention to the needs of the disabled and to practices which, inadvertently or not, have discriminated against them. This initiative contributed to the establishment of both national organizations, such as the Physically Handicapped Association of Nigeria (PHAN) and the Joint National Association of Disabled People (JONADP), and local ones, such as the Disabled Business Association, Kaduna State. The UN Decade for the Disabled initiative has encouraged the Nigerian government and NGOs, as well as disabled groups in Nigeria, to provide programs to assist disabled people as part of the development process. While some state officials have implemented vocational training programs and have helped build workshops to employ disabled people, political instability and economic problems during the 1990s limited the Nigerian government's ability to support programs for the disabled. More recently, however, disabled groups have been demanding (and in some cases receiving) support from federal, state, and local governments, as well as private NGOs, to improve their situation (fig 5.1). These organizations' motivations differ from those of the work carried out by Alhaji Garba in the 1950s. Then, the lame (*guragu*), as a category of people with particular physical conditions, organized themselves into self-help groups with titled chiefs under the patronage of local traditional rulers. During the 1980s, they appear to have recast themselves as citizens who have disabilities and who are entitled to education, vocational training, and support from federal and state governments, as stipulated by the UN initiative.

A result of this international attention to the disabled in Nigeria has been the establishment of programs in different government agencies which are concerned

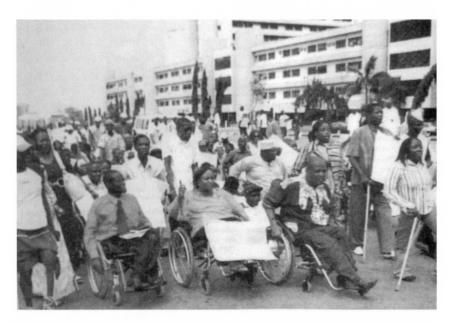

Figure 5.1. Physically disabled members of the Association for Comprehensive Empowerment of Nigerians with Disabilities marching in Abuja in November 2005. The prevalence of wheelchairs and crutches, rather than specially adapted tricycles, suggests that the participants are mainly from southern, rather than northern, Nigeria. *Daily Trust,* 17 November 2005. Photograph by Kennedy Egbomodje, courtesy of the *Daily Trust.*

with the rights of disabled citizens to receive training and assistance. Kaduna State has several programs which benefit the disabled, including a rehabilitation center run by the Kaduna State Rehabilitation Board (established in 1980) as well as special education schools—the Kaduna State Special Education School for the blind and deaf in Kaduna (established in 1979) and the Demonstration School for the Deaf in Kawo (established in 1987)—and a program for mainstreaming disabled students in four secondary schools in Kaduna State (established in 1997–1998)—all three school programs run by the Kaduna State Office of Special Education within the Ministry of Education.

The Kaduna State Rehabilitation Centre

The Kaduna State Rehabilitation Centre Board (RCB) was established to provide training to those with disabilities. The Centre includes a workshop for manufacturing tricycles and other iron products, and also provides training in tailoring, carpentry, shoemaking, weaving and knitting, poultry farming, and animal husbandry to people with a range of disabilities. The main impetus for this training is to reduce begging, as one official with the RCB explained: "Begging has everything to do with work opportunities [and] begging . . . doesn't give a good impression of society" (interview, Kaduna, 22 February 2006).

Along with training, the Centre also provides guidance and assistance to all of the *kungiyar guragu* in the state; each of the twenty-three local government areas has its own organization, and all of these are members of PHAN. The Rehabilitation Centre facilitates communication among these different groups. For example, Centre personnel invited the Kano State branch of PHAN to come to the Centre workshop to discuss the organization of the Kano workshop and to train Kaduna members in making tricycles.

Kaduna State Office of Special Education, Ministry of Education

While the Rehabilitation Centre focuses on providing assistance to disabled associations and vocational training to adults, the Kaduna State Office of Special Education focuses on providing Western education to disabled children. Historically, special education in Nigeria has focused on the blind (Schram 1971, 384–86), with vocational training programs in the 1950s and the establishment of a school for the blind and deaf in Kaduna in 1979. The more recent program for mainstreaming capable disabled students, rather than placing them in special education schools, was instituted in 1997–98 in four secondary schools in Kaduna State (Amwe 2007). Students who have successfully completed six years of primary school are selected on the basis of interviews conducted by the officer in charge of social development at the headquarters of each local government in the state. Candidates are selected by the Ministry of Education Scholarship Board and placed in one of the four schools. The Ministry of Education pays for their food, maintenance, medical costs, examination fees, textbooks, and bedding, while their parents are responsible for uniforms and writing materials. At times, the local government chairmen will also assist disabled students with additional needs (interview, Kaduna, 20 August 2007).

One of the schools participating in the program is Al Huda Huda College in Zaria City. Built in 1910 as a model primary school, it continues to serve both day and boarding students in the area. For disabled students accepted into this program, the government covers their expenses, and they may also be given tricycles to assist them in moving around the spacious campus. According to the school's headmaster, Malam Mohammed Abbas Aliyu, the school admitted forty-four first-year junior and secondary disabled students in the 2006–2007 term, and there were sixty-one disabled students in the school population of approximately two thousand. While physically disabled students generally have little difficulty with schoolwork, a teacher who is himself disabled (he is blind) offers them special support. They are encouraged to participate in sports, and they also have their own association within the school. Despite their excellent educations, some disabled students who graduate from Al Huda Huda have difficulty obtaining employment; as the headmaster noted, "Even those who are [physically] able, they have problems finding jobs." Some parents of disabled children therefore still prefer to have their children beg, despite the changes in thinking about the disabled and the availability of government-subsidized educational opportunities:

Initially they were not many who were wanting to come to school; they might not even worry about going to school. But more recently, disabled people are starting to feel that everyone should be treated as members of society who have the right to go to school . . .

But I believe that there are many [parents] who would prefer begging [bara]. Because they are thinking of immediate results and not thinking of the future. Even those parents who are thinking that at the end of the day [i.e., when they have completed their schooling], they will not find jobs. (Interview, Zaria City, 18 August 2007)

A federal program guarantees that 2 percent of government jobs will be set aside for the disabled, but people do not know about it, and furthermore it is not enforced. Thus the effort to eliminate begging must include efforts to improve expectations and the availability of employment.

The Narrative of a Student with Polio from Zaria

However, one student who completed the program for the disabled at Al Huda Huda College has been successful in obtaining an undergraduate degree and taking up an appointment at a postgraduate institution in Zaria. His experience illustrates changes in explanations for the occurrence of polio, ideas about its treatment, and beliefs about stigma, disability, and begging.

Musa Muhammed was born in 1982 and contracted polio in 1985, when he was three years old. In the early 1980s in Northern Nigeria, vaccines were not always available and public health programs informing parents about the importance of immunization were not widespread. Furthermore, since cases of paralytic polio were uncommon, parents were often not aware of biomedical explanations of this disease. Musa's father, Abdullahi Muhammed, explained his family's initial reaction to his son's illness:

It started from a high fever and he got the sickness when he went to a village with his mother. He was walking and fell down. After one day, he came back to Zaria and at that time, we didn't know it was polio, we thought it was a high fever. When we saw he wasn't walking after three months, they thought it might be Shan Inna. When we realized that we were very sad because my intention was to send Musa to school; I wanted him to be educated. But later my heart was not broken because I could see that he could read. But we suffered to get medicine for him. (Interview, Zaria City, 16 July 2006)

As the family was living in Zaria City, close to the teaching hospital of Ahmadu Bello University and the state hospital at Kofar Gayan, Musa was first taken to these places for treatment. When he did not improve, his father took him to traditional healers (boka) living in villages near Zaria:

I went to one man in Solanke, he is still alive, the woman [healer] is dead. The type of medicine they gave was a salve to put on his legs and a medicine to drink. And they used to do *turare* [medicinal smoke] to be inhaling. They wanted to convince me that it was a spirit that entered his body but I didn't believe them. But honestly, my heart was broken. Even my relatives helped then to get medicine for Musa but I don't know where they got it. They said it was a spirit but I didn't believe them anyway. And I used to take him to ABU for physical therapy for his leg. They put it in one machine, they tried to see if he could walk but he couldn't walk. It took almost three years of going to the hospital that I started thinking [that I shouldn't go with him] to traditional healers or to the hospital. Since we started going looking for medicine, there was no improvement, either in the hospital or with traditional medicine.

We really tried, we looked for medicine, both me and my relatives, and there was even a time when my sister brought medicine and the *turare* they used burnt his leg. ABU was the last place I went for medicine. And I stopped going when he was in primary 3. But before, we went to ABU for physical therapy so he could walk. We even took him to Kano. Since I saw that he was feeling fine and he was going to school, I stopped taking him for medicine.

When he was about seven years old, Musa began to attend primary school in Zaria:

We suffered to take him to school. I would take him on my motorcycle, and if I didn't come in time, his brother would go get him. This was until the time I was able to buy a *keke guragu* [tricycle] for him—he was still in primary school then. At the beginning I was very sad. But we know it was from God, and I want him to read, and he is reading and he has a diploma. (Interview, Zaria City, 16 July 2006)

Because Musa's father was a teacher, he was familiar with the state secondary school program available to the disabled who completed primary school (plate 6). Musa was accepted into this program, which enabled him to attend Al Huda Huda College with government assistance. In 2006, he graduated from Nuhu Bamalli Polytechnic in computer science, after which he performed his Youth Corps service (required of all university graduates in Nigeria) in Kano. He is currently teaching computer science at Nuhu Bamalli Polytechnic.

Musa noted that as a child he had been somewhat ashamed of being physically incapable of doing some things. However, as he gained mobility (first by using a tricycle and later a motorcycle) and an education, he no longer felt ashamed of his disability:

There is a lesson, physical education—so I was feeling that [shame, *abin kunya*], but because I have my bicycle, it reduces that. Now I'm not feeling any shame. You see, the problem is that if the community was feeling that you must feel that, but if they are treating you as everyone else, you won't feel it. . . . No, we don't have that problem, especially if you are going to school. There is that problem only if you are not schooling. (Interview, Zaria, 30 July 2006)

The fact that his father and the general community "treated him as normal" helped him think of himself in this way (interview, Zaria, 8 July 2005).

COMPASS, the Polio-Disabled, and the Polio Eradication Initiative

As well as the programs aimed at providing disabled people with secondary and postsecondary education, there are vocational training programs, mainly for adults, teaching trades in which the expectations of immediate income are somewhat greater (Aodu 2007a). In Kaduna State and in other Northern Nigerian states, NGOs such as the International Red Cross and COMPASS sponsor or support several such programs. Rotary International is indirectly involved through the actions of individual members, such as the Rotarian owner of Rainbow Nursery and Primary School in Hotoro, Kano, who allows polio-disabled children to attend his school for reduced fees (Owens-Ibie 2005).[9] The involvement of Rotary members and of COMPASS personnel in assisting the physically disabled is related to Rotary International's and USAID's involvement in the Polio Eradication Initiative.

The COMPASS program (which ended in 2009) was discussed in chapter 3 in the context of the 2006 reorganization of the Polio Eradication Initiative. By working with community political and religious leaders as well as with community health workers and the polio-disabled in local communities, COMPASS personnel attempted to integrate public health interventions with local perspectives and needs. The COMPASS program helped to plan polio immunization activities and evaluation, to identify children under five with acute flaccid paralysis, and to involve polio-disabled people in the 2006 Immunization Plus Days (COMPASS 2007a; Walker 2007a). COMPASS personnel also provided training and microcredit funds to the polio-disabled. Most of this rehabilitation work was carried out in Kano, and it has involved several members of the Kano Polio Victims Trust Association, which was organized in 1990 (Owens-Ibie 2005). This Kano-based group is particularly well organized and has supported vocational training at a workshop making tricycles for the lame (*keke guragu;* plate 7) which it sells along a main road in Kano. In 2005, it raised funds to educate eighty-five disabled children to the secondary school level. The group paid for their school uniforms and books, and prevailed upon school headmasters and principals to defray their school fees (interview, Kano, 26 August 2005). The Kano Polio Victims Trust Association also provides adult education for its members.

In its turn, the Kano State government has responded to the demands of the disabled by appointing a special advisor, Alhaji Safiyanu Ado, who is himself disabled and a member of the Kano Polio Victims Trust Association. The governor of Kano State, Ibrahim Shekarau, has promised "to offer free education to all disabled pupils in public schools" (Kwaru 2007). In addition, he has also provided financial support for a census of the disabled in Kano in order to assess their needs and to reduce begging,[10] much as was done by the colonial government in Ghana in the 1950s. It is also possible that the new view of disability as a problem which can be remedied, and of begging as shameful not only for those who practice it but for societies which countenance it by not providing alternatives, will itself reduce the incidence of begging in the twenty-first century in Kano and Kaduna States.

* * *

> So long as cripples are to be found all over the place,
> And blind, both men and women,
> Having no proper place in all Hausa country,
> No one to aid them with his wealth,
> So that they wander in city and villages
> And through all the towns of Nigeria—
> *Kai*! The Hausa has no heart
> And he will face the world with shame![11]

— Sa'adu Zungur, The North, Republic or Monarchy?
poem quoted in Furniss, Poetry, Prose and Popular Culture in Hausa

Those with physical disabilities in Northern Nigeria live within changing political, economic, and sociocultural contexts. The early attribution of paralysis and subsequent lameness to spirits fostered an image of the polio-disabled as helpless and incapable and of begging as their only option. While conversion to Islam changed lameness from something caused by spirits to something from Allah, the disabled continued to beg as part of a system of alms-giving and mendicancy. Government efforts, at least on paper, to provide rehabilitative training for the disabled in order to reduce begging began during the colonial period. These efforts have continued intermittently since Independence. With the UN declaration of the Decade of the Disabled, more federal and state governments, as well as NGOs, have introduced programs for training and Western education. While the impact of these programs on the lives of the polio-disabled in Northern Nigeria is not known, the messages that these programs are promoting—that one can overcome disability with education, that income-generating work is preferable to begging, that begging is not an inherent aspect of Islam, and that the disabled should join together to assert their right to government assistance—have influenced people's thinking, particularly that of the young.

The excerpt from a poem by Sa'adu Zungur, a Hausa poet and political activist, quoted above captures this increasing disapproval of public begging in Northern Nigeria and argues that the practice reveals the Hausa people as backward and heartless. Yet efforts to eliminate begging, like those to eradicate polio, reflect specific economic situations, and inequality leads some to respond to such efforts in particular ways. Thus people disabled by polio in Zaria City who came from well-to-do families pursued Western education and did not beg, while those without these advantages attended Islamic schools and did. Similarly, some people have benefited from the various rehabilitative and education schemes, although whether they beg is determined as much by their socioeconomic backgrounds as by such schemes. However, the existence of these programs and the reassessment of begging by young Hausa men and women, who see it as not only shameful but also un-Islamic, along with an improvement in the economy, may lead to a

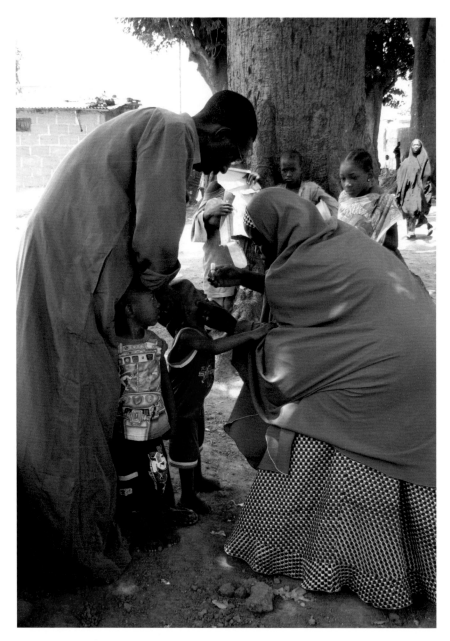

Plate 1. Health worker giving drops of oral polio vaccine to a child during a Sub-National Immunization Day exercise in Zaria City. *Photograph by E. P. Renne, 2 June 2009.*

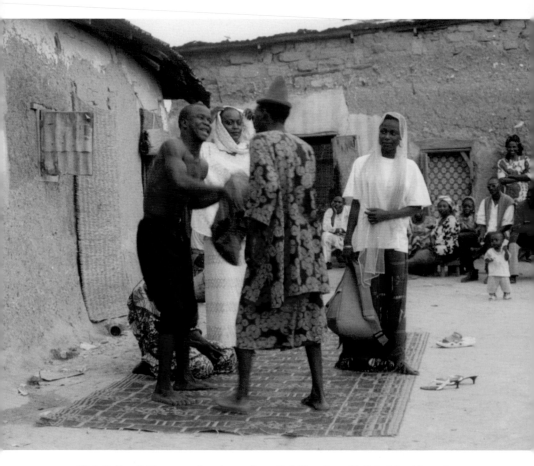

Plate 2. Gamji Players performing a play called *Shan Inna* (Polio). A health worker attempts to enter a house to administer the oral polio vaccine but is stopped by the child's father. The child is subsequently paralyzed by polio. The small boy standing offstage to the back right was incorporated into the performance. *Photograph by E. P. Renne, Samaru, 20 July 2005.*

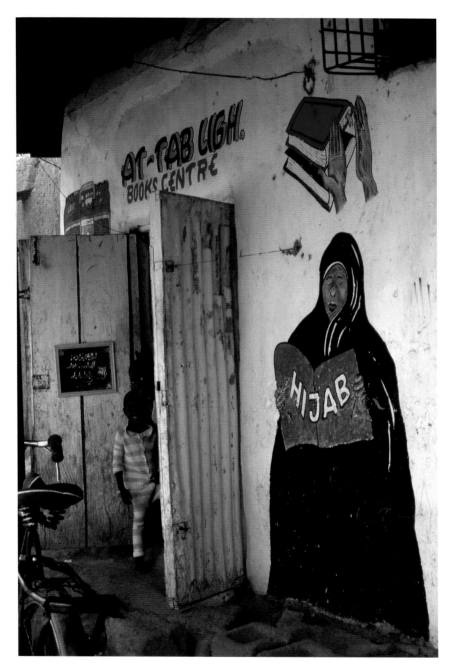

Plate 3. Painting advertising a bookshop specializing in Islamic literature along the main road to the market in Zaria City. A woman is depicted both wearing a hijab and reading a book titled *Hijab,* which refers to the expansion of Islamic education for married women, beginning in the 1970s. *Photograph by E. P. Renne, Zaria City, 1996.*

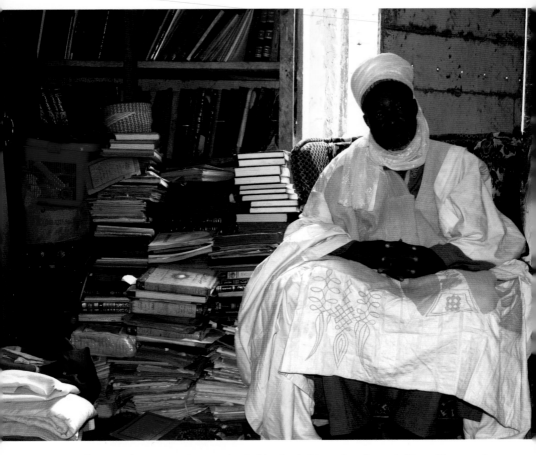

Plate 4. Malam Husseini, a popular Sufi healer, in his study at home in Kano. *Photograph by E. P. Renne, Kano, 23 July 2006.*

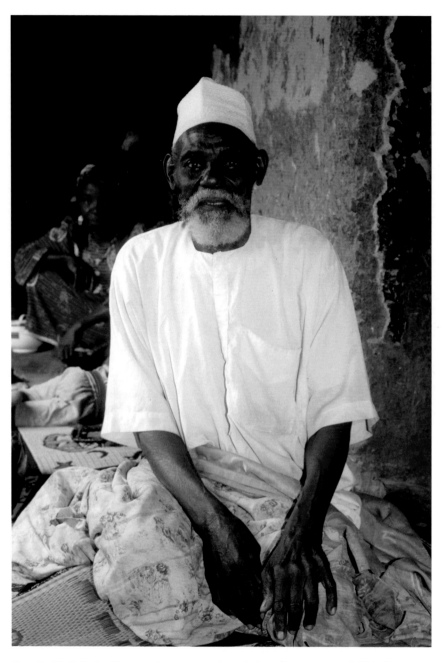

Plate 5. Alhaji Garba Hassan, who contracted paralytic polio as a young child in Zaria, traveled throughout West Africa helping to organize associations for the lame. *Photograph by E. P. Renne, Yakasai, August 2005.*

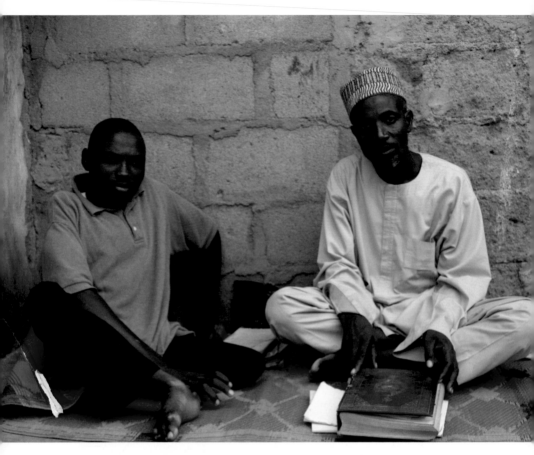

Plate 6. Malam Abdullahi Muhammed and his son, Musa Muhammed, at home in Anguwar Jussi. Musa Muhammed was paralyzed by polio when he was three years old in 1985. Through his father's efforts and his own initiative, he obtained an education and is now teaching computer science at Nuhu Bamalli Polytechnic. *Photograph by E. P. Renne, Zaria City, 16 July 2006.*

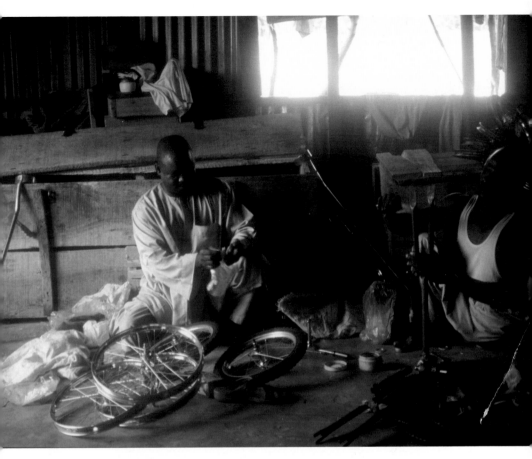

Plate 7. Two physically disabled workers at the Kano Polio Victims Trust Association (a member of PHAN, the Physically Handicapped Association of Nigeria) workshop in Kano, constructing tricycles (*keke guragu*) designed for those whose legs have been paralyzed by polio. *Photograph by E. P. Renne, Kano, August 2005.*

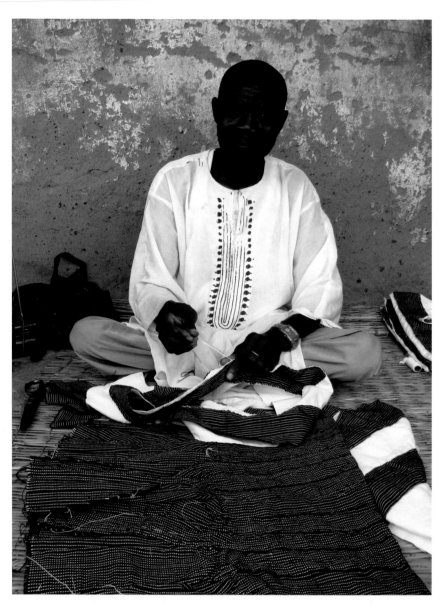

Plate 8. Shirazu Moru was born in the mid-1970s and contracted polio when he was about one year old; childhood vaccinations were not routinely provided at that time. His parents took him to the Yendi Hospital in northeastern Ghana, where he was given injections, after which he became paralyzed in both legs. Despite his disability, his parents supported him through primary school, although he stopped attending school after their deaths. He was later sent to the University of Ghana Teaching Hospital at Korle Bu for nine months of physical therapy. He now works as a tailor, sewing handwoven cloth strips together to construct the smocks for which the Dagomba are famous, and he regularly takes his daughter for vaccinations during National Immunization Days.
Photograph by E. P. Renne, Yendi, May 2009.

reduction of public begging in Northern Nigeria. These distinctive responses of the polio-disabled to begging in the North further accentuate the differences in the life experiences of those who have been affected by paralytic polio. The variable extent to which these different life experiences may be improved by government and NGO programs is paralleled by the variable effectiveness of national polio eradication and immunization strategies, as may be seen in a comparison of programs implemented in Ghana and Nigeria.

6. Polio in Northern Nigeria and Northeastern Ghana

President Umaru Musa Yar'adua has promised Nigerians and the international community of his administration's commitment to stem the further transmission of polio virus and make Nigeria a polio-free country.

—*Daily Trust,* 29 March 2009

Barely a year after World Health Organisation (WHO) declared Ghana polio free, a positive polio case has been detected at Yendi Hospital, medical doctors confirmed to GNA on Friday.

—Ghana News Agency, "Polio case detected in Yendi"

As these news reports from Nigeria and Ghana suggest, the Polio Eradication Initiative has met with variable success in West Africa. In Ghana, with its well-organized program of routine immunization and high levels of immunization overall, there were no wild poliovirus infections between 2004 and 2007, although eight cases of polio were confirmed in 2008. In Nigeria, there have been no such breaks in polio transmission, although in 2006, with the implementation of Immunization Plus Days, the total number of cases had declined considerably (see chapter 3). Yet by the end of 2008, the number of confirmed cases of wild poliovirus in Nigeria had almost tripled.[1] Additionally, several countries in West Africa—Benin, Burkina Faso, Côte d'Ivoire, Mali, Niger, and Togo, as well as Ghana—reported cases which, when analyzed using genomic sequencing, were found to have originated in Northern Nigeria (CDC 2009c, 309). How can these increases be explained, and how have poliovirus strains from Northern Nigeria traveled to Northeastern Ghana? Furthermore, how have migration and identity, which may be matters of ethnicity and religion rather than of allegiance to a particular nation-state, affected the Polio Eradication Initiative's efforts, which in West Africa are organized by national programs?

Taxis and buses carry Hausa traders and businessmen along a network of roads that connect Northern Nigeria with Niger, Chad, Benin, Burkina Faso, Côte d'Ivoire, Ghana, Mali, and Togo. Many of these men have family and work connections with others living both within and outside of Nigeria. These men, who may at times bring their wives and children with them, may carry the wild poliovirus with them as well. Additionally, migratory Fulani families, who travel with their cattle, frequently cross the Nigeria-Niger border. In Northeastern Ghana and Togo, several ethnic groups straddle national boundaries, with family members traveling back and forth on a regular basis. The children of these mobile populations may or may not have received the oral polio vaccine, depending on where they were at the time that a particular National Immunization Day was held. In 2009, health officials addressed these transnational flows of people and polio by synchronizing National Immunization Days in West Africa, as had been done through 2005 (see table 3.1). However, the effectiveness of state and local programs for routine immunization has also affected the prevalence of polio in Nigeria and Ghana. How does the availability of vaccines and primary health care contribute to and help to explain the distinctive responses of parents living in Northern Nigeria and Northeastern Ghana to the Polio Eradication Initiative?

While the variable successes of these programs reflect these governments' commitment—both in theory and in practice—to the Polio Eradication Initiative, they also reflect the distinctive social, cultural, historical, and political contexts of the areas of Northern Nigeria and Northeastern Ghana where the majority of polio cases have occurred. An examination of these contexts and of parents' experiences and understandings of *gbalibila fiep-fiep* ("lame leg"), as it is called by the Dagomba of Yendi District in the Northern Region of Northeastern Ghana, helps to explain why parents respond as they do to government efforts to eradicate polio, and why the responses of some parents in Northern Nigeria differed from those of parents in Northeastern Ghana. It also helps to explain why from 2001 to 2008 Ghana had only sixteen confirmed cases of wild poliovirus while Nigeria had 4,372, and why the 2008 outbreak in Ghana occurred only in the Northern Region.

A comparison of polio in the Northern Region of Ghana and in Northern Nigeria is instructive, as they are similar in several ways. Both areas are predominantly Muslim,[2] have largely agricultural populations, and retain forms of traditional political organization distinguished by royal families and commoners, whose histories are entangled with British colonial rule (Lentz 2006; Miles 1994). Furthermore, local medical practices continue to be used (and to be preferred by some) alongside various forms of Western medicine (Bierlich 2000, 2007; M. Last 2004; Wall 1988). Yet while there has been some resistance to routine immunization and to the Polio Eradication Initiative in the Northern Region—in 2003, it had the lowest levels of overall childhood immunization in Ghana (Ghana Statistical Service, Noguchi Memorial Institute for Medical Research, and ORC Macro 2004, 154)[3]— this resistance is based on culturally specific interpretations of vaccines and on particular political preoccupations. In Ghana, there have not been widespread rumors linking the Polio Eradication Initiative to infertility, although people in the Northern Region heard news of the polio vaccination boycott in Northern Nigeria. Furthermore, in Yendi, the capital of Yendi District in the Northern Region, the Muslim community actively participated in the Polio Eradication Initiative, announcing National Immunization Days in Friday mosque services and allowing immunizations in Islamic schools. This participation is indicative of the difference between Islamic attitudes and practices there and those in many parts of Northern Nigeria. Nor have there been long periods of time when vaccines were unavailable (as they were in Nigeria in early 2006). The Ghanaian government's involvement in statewide primary health care programs, particularly routine immunization, and its provision of basic infrastructure has promoted public cooperation with and even trust of government efforts, which has affected people's experiences of polio immunization as well as their reception of their government's involvement in the polio campaign.

Explanations of the Oral Polio Vaccine and Paralysis in Yendi District

The initial responses of people in the Northern Region, especially in Yendi District, where the majority of my interviews took place, were not altogether different from those of parents in Zaria, in Northern Nigeria. Rather, they present variations on common themes, which include distrust, ambivalence, and fear as well as acceptance. For instance, the belief that vaccines contain antifertility substances has arisen in both Zaria and Yendi, although in Zaria, it was the oral polio vaccine that was the focus of distrust, while in Yendi District it was tetanus toxoid vaccine (given to pregnant mothers during a campaign to reduce neonatal tetanus) that was suspect (interview, Yendi, 23 May 2009).

Similarly, beliefs about the consequences of the oral polio vaccine also differ. While parents in Zaria who refused to allow their children to be vaccinated did so out of fears for the future, those who accepted the vaccine had no complaints of side effects, although a few parents whose children contracted polio after having taken the vaccine believed that it had caused their children's paralysis. However, in Yendi, there was a widespread perception that the polio vaccine caused diarrhea, which led some to avoid vaccinating their children:

> People believe that when they immunize their children, they run diarrhea. Even the health workers are aware [of this]. They have fever so because of that, some may not want to immunize their children. . . . When they come to the house, they may run away with their children. (Interview, Yendi, 21 May 2009)

One health officer suggested that the diarrhea was caused by community volunteers engaged in the house-to-house polio vaccination campaign who gave larger doses that were required:

> EPR: That fear of diarrhea, is it from injections or the drops or both?
> MF: Polio, the oral one, but the injectibles, no—just the oral polio one. We even experienced it during this campaign. We don't entirely use health staff, we use volunteers, both to help in reaching all the eligible children. In so doing there is bound to be some overdosing somehow, and in that, perhaps, may result in diarrhea. But with the routine [immunization], we don't experience it at all. (Interview, Yendi, 23 May 2009)

While it is unclear precisely why these children experienced diarrhea, such occurrences reinforce parents' unease about their children's ingesting an unknown substance associated with powerful Western medicine (Bierlich 2000).

Indeed, the views of parents in Yendi and Zaria regarding one form of Western medicine—the injection—tend to converge. As was discussed in chapter 4, injections have been widely accepted as a potent source of healing in West Africa, but may also be seen as dangerous. Bierlich, who worked in the Northern Region in the early 1990s, notes that "injection-therapy (one of the most powerful exponents of biomedicine) occupies an ambiguous position in people's minds because of it being not only powerful but also foreign and not attuned to local notions and practices of dealing with illness" (2000, 710). According to local logic, an injection forces the disease to come out. In the case of fever—a symptom of both malaria and polio—this is good; the fever will come out and disappear. But in the case of polio, whose defining symptom is paralysis, an injection will cause a child to become paralyzed, as one health worker explained:

> You see, . . . when the disease [doesn't] manifest itself, the medical officers can test to see if the child has the disease, you understand? But you don't [necessarily] see the disease in the form of maiming. But immediately the person will get an injection, the disease will come out. So, in fact, it took a very long time to convince people . . . that it was not the injection that was doing that . . . as a lot of people believed if you were injected you would become lame. It was then, but now, they don't think that. (Interview, Yendi, 21 May 2009)

In Yendi, the fear that injections may cause paralysis has impeded measles vaccination efforts, although, according to this health worker, this belief has been largely dispelled. In Northern Nigeria, some traditional healers, such as the healer in Solanke outside of Zaria, continue to attribute paralysis to medical doctors' indiscriminate use of injections.

These sometimes different and sometimes overlapping interpretations of vaccines and injections reflect parents' common concerns for their children's health. They wish to cure illness but are wary of powerful foreign medicines. These twin concerns for cure and caution are apparent in the cases of polio that occurred in Yendi District in 2003 and 2008.[4]

Of the three confirmed cases of polio that occurred in the Northern Region in 2003, one case was identified in Kpunkpano, a village along the Yendi-Bimbilla road in Yendi District. The child's mother had run away with her child to another village to avoid vaccination. (It is possible that she feared the side effects of the vaccine; she was variously described as "afraid" and as "stubborn.") When the child became paralyzed she returned to Kpunkpano, where health officials confirmed that the child had polio (interview, 21 May 2009, Yendi).

Five years later, two cases were also reported in Yendi District. The first was a two-year-old girl living with her parents in a village west of Yendi along the main Yendi-Tamale road. According to one district health officer, the girl's health card showed that she had received the complete course of childhood immunizations, including polio vaccine, at the local health clinic. On 8 September 2008, she developed a fever, although there was no vomiting or diarrhea. Her parents bought a multivitamin supplement and malaria medicine at a local drug store, but her health did not improve. Her mother then brought her to the Yendi Hospital, where she was admitted to the children's ward, diagnosed with malaria, and treated. However, when lab tests for malaria were negative, the doctor noticed some paralysis of the girl's legs. The disease control officer was notified, and stool samples were taken and sent to Tamale, the capital of the Northern Region. Analysis of the samples confirmed that the girl had contracted type 1 poliovirus (interview, Yendi, 23 May 2009).

There are a number of puzzling things about this case. Not only had the girl been fully immunized, but her parents had participated in National Immunization Days as well. None of her six siblings had symptoms of the disease and neither she nor her parents, who were farmers, had left their village. It is still unclear precisely why the child did not develop immunity after receiving numerous doses of polio vaccine, although it is possible that she was already infected with competing enteroviruses which prevented her from acquiring immunity.

The second case, a four-year-old boy living with his mother in Yendi town who became ill in mid-October, was less mysterious, as there was no evidence that he had received the full sequence of polio vaccinations, and may not have received any at all. His mother, a trader who had traveled to Accra, had left the boy with his grandmother in Tamale. Upon the grandmother's death, the mother returned and took her son with her to Yendi. On 17 October 2008, the child developed a fever and was unable to stand or walk. At Yendi Hospital he was diagnosed—because of the fever—as having severe malaria and was admitted. He subsequently received treatment for malaria, including three quinine injections, along with paracetamol. However, continued weakness in his legs led the hospital staff to request that stool samples be taken on 22 October, which proved to be positive for polio. A control officer explained this case as caused by irresponsibility, rather than by fear of immunization or of vaccine failure:

> Yes, she [the mother] didn't have time to send the child for immunization, so the child had no records at all. So that one came as a positive case, we weren't really surprised. We took the stool samples, the immunization records were just not there. And the history of immunization for NIDs, you know . . . we don't have any documentation to prove [it], we are just going around [giving vaccine]. (Interview, Yendi, 23 May 2009)

These three cases exemplify three different responses to routine immunization and the polio campaign in Yendi District: fear, compliance, and indifference. Furthermore, while education programs aim to tell people about the possible side effects of vaccination and health incentives encourage people to immunize their children, the fact that in rare instances children who have received four doses (or more) of polio vaccine still contract polio complicates these efforts. Despite the difficulties of achieving high levels of immunization, these efforts have been relatively effective in Ghana as compared with Nigeria, reflecting differences in the administration and conduct of immunization programs and distinctive political concerns.

Comparing Immunization Programs in Ghana and Nigeria

While the two countries differ in landmass and population—in 2007 Ghana had a population of 23,478,000, Nigeria 148,093,000 (UNICEF 2009), these differences cannot entirely explain why Ghana was twice able to become polio-free for some time, while wild poliovirus continues to be endemic in Nigeria. In Ghana, overall high levels of routine immunization for early childhood diseases, consistent eradication efforts at the federal and regional levels, and a general acceptance of a national program of immunization have contributed to the success of the Ghanaian polio eradication program. However, factors similar to those in Northern Nigeria contributed to the recurrence of cases in Ghana's Northern Region in 2003 and 2008. Like Northern Nigeria, the Northern Region of Ghana accounts for a large part of the country; the Northern Region occupies approximately one-third of Ghana's landmass. The difficulty of reaching its dispersed communities and the relative dearth of health workers have hindered immunization efforts there. Also, Western education came late to this area, as it did to Northern Nigeria. One man explained, "If you take all of us, those of us from a Muslim home or community, our education came to us by accident because we come from a community that doesn't believe in secular or Western ideas, including their health care, education, and so on" (interview, Yendi, 21 May 2009). Some health workers see this lag (and, for some, disinterest in Western education) as hampering their efforts to explain the health benefits of immunization; people "have their own perceptions, especially in the Northern [Region]," observed one health official (interview, Yendi, 23 May 2009). One might also say that they have their own perceptions of how Western biomedicine relates to local understandings of health and medical practice (Bierlich 2007).

One person I interviewed described the Northern Region as the most politically unstable area of the country. Its numerous ethnic and chieftaincy disputes have at times impeded National Immunization Day activities and have contributed to distrust of oral polio vaccine. For example, a dispute over chieftainship of the town of Wenchiki led health workers to cancel Immunization Day activities in the Chereponi District in January 2009 (interview, Tamale, 22 May 2009). But these difficulties are not the same as the resistance specifically to the Polio Eradication Initiative that is found in Northern Nigeria. There, resistance has functioned as a way to express discontent with the government's failure to provide basic health services and with the Initiative's focus on polio. The Initiative is also resisted because it is associated with the West. Thus, while some factors contributing to the 2008 polio outbreak in the Northern Region are similar to ones operating in Northern Nigeria, others are specific to Ghana. Immunization programs in the two countries are run differently, and their citizens have different conceptions of their relationship to an international Muslim community. Lastly, expectations of adequate health care, including the availability of childhood vaccines free of charge, have been differently met by the various immunization programs.

The National Expanded Programme on Immunisation in Ghana

In Ghana, the Expanded Programme on Immunisation, which was implemented in 1996 by the Ministry of Health, supports routine immunization, control and surveillance of vaccine-preventable diseases, cold chain and vaccine management, and injection safety and waste management (WHO Ghana 2003). In 1998, Ghana Health Service officials reorganized the Programme under the newly formed Inter-Agency Coordinating Committee in order to improve its operations, financial oversight, and applications for funding. Although the Programme's budget for vaccines and immunization implementation has come mainly from NGOs and foreign donors,[5] the enormous national debt which had accumulated by 2000 led government leaders to apply for assistance through the Heavily Indebted Poor Country Initiative (a joint project of the IMF and the World Bank) in 2001 (WHO Ghana 2003). After qualifying for debt relief and receiving funding from the Gates Foundation's Global Alliance for Vaccines and Immunization, the government increased its support of health programs, including routine immunization. The success of these efforts is evident in the rising overall immunization levels of children between twelve and twenty-three months old, from 47 percent in 1988 to 69 percent in 2003 (Ghana Statistical Service, Noguchi Memorial Institute for Medical Research, and ORC Macro 2004). Overall immunization levels of children the same age in Nigeria in 2003 were 13 percent (National Population Commission and ORC Macro 2004, 130). These disparities in immunization levels have continued into 2007, with Ghanaian and Nigerian tuberculosis vaccination rates at 99 percent and 69 percent, measles vaccination at 95 percent and 62 percent, and polio vaccination (three doses) at 94 percent and 61 percent, respectively (UNICEF 2009).

The considerable difference in national levels of polio immunization in Ghana and Nigeria reflect differences in program operations. The Nigerian National Programme on Immunization has experienced vaccine shortages and discontinuities in leadership (see chapter 3), while the Ghanaian Expanded Programme on Immunisation has had a steady supply of vaccine and personnel continuity at the national, state, and local levels. Thus Dr. Kwadwo Antwi Agyei has headed the National Expanded Programme on Immunisation since 2003, and in the Northern Region both the director of public health and the regional manager of the Expanded Programme on Immunisation have worked with the Programme since 1996.

National Immunization Days and Responses to the 2008 Polio Outbreak

In response to the 2008 outbreak, the Ghana Health Service organized National Immunization Day rounds in October and November 2008. Health workers went house to house with doses of oral polio vaccine in order to improve coverage of all children under the age of five.[6] House-to-house vaccination, which had been stopped in 2005 (interview, Tamale, 22 May 2009), was reinstituted in order to find children who had not received routine immunization at local clinics and hospitals.

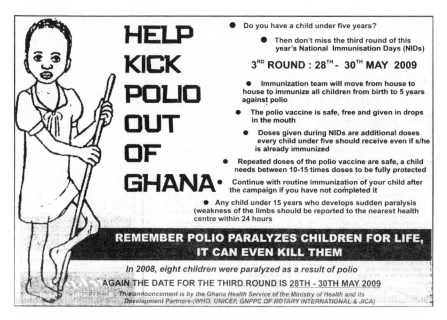

Figure 6.1. Advertisement for the upcoming third round of National Immunisation Days exercises (28–30 May 2009), published in the *Daily Graphic*, 23 May 2009. One community health worker from Madina-Zongo (in Accra) noted that few people would see such newspaper advertisements, because papers were prohibitively expensive. Courtesy of the Ghana Health Service, EPI Programme.

To further reduce the possibility of a resurgence of cases in 2009, house-to-house National Immunization Day rounds were also conducted in February and March 2009. Dr. Antwi Agyei explained in February how they would be carried out:

> Some 42,500 volunteers would move from house-to-house throughout the country to carry out the exercise. The NIDs will have Vitamin A being given to 3.3 million children from six months to five years. . . . He explained that the doses that would be given to targeted children during the NIDs would be extra doses of polio vaccines that every child under-five years should receive even if the child had already been immunized. It does not replace routine immunization. (Ghana News Agency 2009)

Additionally, on 28–30 May 2009, Ghanaian health workers participated in synchronized National Immunization Days that took place across West Africa in order to stop the regional spread of polio (fig. 6.1). To date, they have been successful in their efforts, with no cases reported as of 11 December 2009, even as their neighbors to the north, east, and west continue to report them. Nonetheless, the difficulties confronting health personnel in the Northern Region have complicated their task.[7]

Polio and Politics in the Northern Region

There is a dearth of accessible health services and health workers in the Northern Region, as a result of its geography, population mobility, budgetary constraints, and political factors. Aside from Tamale, the Region's capital, only two health centers—in Yendi and Bimbilla—are headed by permanent medical doctors. Other hospitals and clinics rely on volunteer doctors from the Cuban Medical Brigade, when available. At times, medical technicians, who may not have adequate training, manage local hospitals and clinics. This situation has historical precedents, for during the early independence period it was difficult to provide doctors for the health centers in Yendi District and vaccines were not regularly available (plate 8). In August 1966 the Yendi Hospital's resident doctor, who was on leave, was "called to Tamale for an indefinite period of time." He was still absent in November 1967, when the district administrative officer, J. E. Nsaful, wrote,

> The Yendi Hospital has been without a Medical Officer for sometime now and a Ward Master has been acting in the place of a Doctor. The position is not encouraging. The Health Centres at Bimbilla and Chereponi should be served by the Medical Officer stationed at Yendi so that with the absence of a Doctor at the Yendi Hospital, both the Yendi and Bimbilla Districts are uncared for. The several empty beds do not reflect the state of the people's health but rather lack of confidence.

However, in early December 1967, Nsaful reported that a doctor had at last been appointed (Nsaful 1967).

Other factors have also affected the availability of medical staff in Yendi. In March 2002, political violence between two royal families over the selection, installation, and burial of the Dagomba *ya na* (king) led many medical staff to leave the area:

> The only hospital in Yendi is the Yendi District Hospital. Before March 2002, this hospital had one Ghanaian doctor assisted by four Cuban doctors. On the 27th March, the Cuban Embassy in Accra sent a rescue team to pick up their doctors leaving the District Health Director as the only doctor in the hospital, assisted by understaffed nurses. . . . According to the Principal Nursing Officer and the Executive Director of the hospital, there were about fifty nurses in the hospital before the 2002 conflict. Immediately after the conflict, some of the nurses did not come back and others only returned to collect their release letters. (Anamzoya 2004, 174)

While some secondary school graduates were trained to serve as ward assistants, they were in fact acting as nurses, with the remaining nurses acting as doctors. During this period, "the Yendi hospital [was seen] as a death trap," although this situation was remedied by the placement of two Cuban doctors at the hospital in 2004 (Anamzoya 2004, 174). The bloodshed of March 2002 and the fear it engendered also disrupted routine immunization efforts in Yendi.

Ethnic Conflicts in the Northern Region

As well as the political violence in Yendi, clashes between the many ethnic groups in the Northern Region—the Dagomba, Konkomba, Mamprussi, Gonja,

Nawri, Nanumba, Basari, and Anufo—mainly over land, political authority, and ethnic autonomy, have also affected polio eradication efforts. For example, ethnic disputes between the majority Dagomba and minority Konkomba in Yendi District have contributed to fears of vaccination, particularly when the ethnicity of vaccination team members differs from that of children's parents. Thus in 1996, when a Dagomba health worker went to the town of Zabzugu, in Zabzugu-Tatale District, as part of a polio immunization team, Konkomba parents there refused to let him immunize their children unless he first took a drop himself of every dose that he gave to them—which he did (interview, Accra, 19 May 2009).[8]

Like Yendi and Zabzugu-Tatale Districts, two other districts—East and West Mamprussi—have also been subject to ethnic violence;[9] these four districts accounted for five of the eight cases of poliovirus in 2008. In all of the confirmed cases, subsequent genomic sequencing of the poliovirus samples confirmed a wild poliovirus of Northern Nigerian origin (CDC 2009a). In the two cases from Yendi District, however, neither the children nor their parents had traveled out of Ghana, raising the question of how they could have contracted a strain of the virus traced to Northern Nigeria.

People's Networks: Roads, Cattle, and Radios

While West Africa is divided by national boundaries, these boundaries do not always coincide with ethnic boundaries which, while more amorphous, may transcend the national boundaries drawn on maps (Miles 1994). Thus Hausa people in Northern Nigeria and southern Niger may have families living in Kano and Maradi, and relatives may frequently travel between these two areas (Cooper 1997).[10] Similarly, in Northeastern Ghana, there are ethnic groups whose family and work connections transcend the cartological line that divides them, as one man living in Yendi explained:

> Because you take Togo, for instance, if you take the Northern Region crossing the border, you can count up to three ethnic groups or more who are divided. Some are in Togo, some are in the Northern Region. Kolokoli is one, the Konkombas are one, the Basari, and the Anufos. . . . If you take the Anufo, for instance, if you take Charcole, which happens to be their biggest settlement in Ghana, then their largest settlement in Togo is called [Sansanné-]Mango—and people commute [back and forth], day in day out. . . . Even in my family house, I mean living here, there are people with families who are based in Togo. When they vacate [the house], they go to Togo, and some from Togo go to Ghana. (Interview, Yendi, 21 May 2009)[11]

These overlapping ethnic and family relationships illustrate a sort of transitive property of polio. Infants and children who have asymptomatic cases of the disease may travel with their families to one town and spread the disease through their feces, which infects children from this town who may travel to another, and so on. As one Kano taxi driver who regularly traveled to Maradi, Niger, explained, a trader may bring his family with him from Maradi to Kano, stay for some time to conduct business, and then later return with them to Maradi (interview, Kano, 10 June 2009). Other families may travel westward from Maradi through Niger and Burkina Faso, and then south through Togo to Sansanné-Mango and Bassari, where the road westward leads to Zabzugu, Yendi, and Tamale. Additionally, people from Sokoto and from Birnin Kebbi in Kebbi State, where polio cases were confirmed in 2008, may travel westward through the border town of Gaya to Kamba and Kandi in Benin, then on to Sokodé and Bassari in Togo, and from there to Zabzugu-Tatale and Yendi in Ghana. Alternatively, they may follow the old route taken by Alhaji Garba in the 1950s (see map 5.1), from Zaria to Lagos and then through Cotonou (Benin), Lomé (Togo), and on to Accra (Ghana). Since the poliovirus can live outside the human body, e.g., in open sewers, for three months or more, its transmission may continue over an extended period of time (Polio Information Center Online 2002).

The impact of these road connections may be seen in the distribution of confirmed cases of polio in Ghana, with many cases occurring along routes plied by taxis and buses coming from Burkina Faso, Togo, and Benin, as well as indirectly from Niger and Northern Nigeria (map 6.1). In Ghana, these include cases in Zabzugu-Tatale, Yendi, and Savelugu-Nanton Districts, all which are transected by or border the main road from Togo to Tamale. Three more cases were identified in East Mamprussi, Gushegu, and Tolon-Kunbungu Districts, along with one unconfirmed case in West Mamprussi District, which are linked by roads emanating out of Yendi to the north and Tamale to the west.

In addition to being spread by travelers on taxis and buses, the poliovirus may also be spread by migratory populations, such as Fulani herdsmen and their families. Because they follow their cattle as they graze and follow "bush paths," rather than roads, which may cross national borders, they are not associated with specific local government clinics, nor are they easily located during National Immunization Days and at official border check-points. Thus the immunization director of Kebbi State blamed an outbreak of polio in Birnin Kebbi, in northeastern Nigeria, on Fulani migrants (H. Muhammad 2009), although it is unclear precisely how this attribution was determined. While in this instance poliovirus spread within Nigeria itself, Fulani groups frequently move between Nigeria and Niger, so they may indeed contribute to the spread of polio to neighboring countries.

WHO and CDC health officials, along with their counterparts in the national health ministry, are well aware of the transnational mobility of those whom they seek to immunize.[12] Yet because the Polio Eradication Initiative is organized independently in each nation-state, the problems posed by this mobility are addressed only imperfectly, by synchronizing National Immunization Days, with immunization teams also present at major border crossings during these days. Synchronized National Immunization Days were carried out in West Africa in 2004 and 2005, and after the outbreak of cases in Ghana, Togo, Benin, and Burkina Faso in 2008 and continuing new cases in 2009, a coordinated program of National Immunization Days was staged in Ghana, Togo, Niger (28–30 May), Nigeria (30 May–2 June), and Benin (three weeks later, as a result of a health workers' strike; see table 3.1).

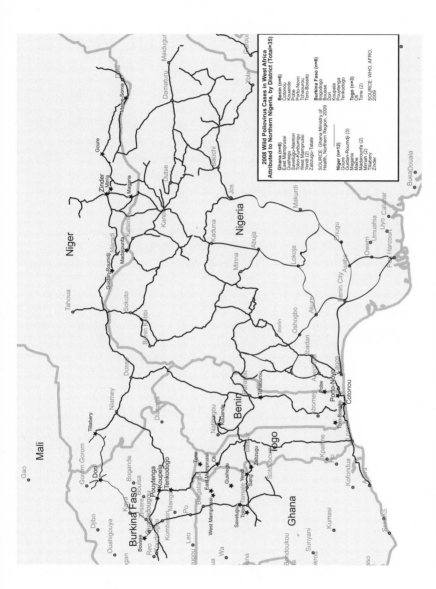

2008 Wild Poliovirus Cases in West Africa Attributed to Northern Nigeria, by District (Total=35)

Ghana (n=8)	**Benin (n=6)**
East Mamprussi	Cotonou
Gushegu	Kouande
Savelugu–Nanton	Pobe
Tolon–Kunbumgu	Porto-Novo
West Mamprussi	Tchaourou
Yendi (2)	Toro-Bossito
Zabzugu–Tatale	
	Burkina Faso (n=6)
SOURCE: Ghana Ministry of	Bogodogo
Health, Northern Region, 2009	Boussé
	Dori
	Koupela
Niger (n=12)	Pouytenga
Guidan-Roumdji (3)	Tenkodogo
Magaria	
Maine	**Togo (n=3)**
Madarounfa (2)	Oti
Mirriah (2)	Tone (2)
Tillabery	
Zinder	SOURCE: WHO, AFRO,
	2009

Map 6.1. Map of West Africa, showing roads from Northern Nigeria to Niger, Benin, Burkina Faso, Togo, and the Northern Region of Ghana. In 2008, confirmed cases of polio were reported in the districts of Magaria, Zinder, Gouré, Guidan-Roumdji, and Tillabery (Niger); Dori (Burkina Faso); Tchaourou (Benin); Sansanné-Mango (Togo); and Yendi and Zabzugu (Ghana).

In Ghana, a considerable effort has been made to immunize children at border towns and at major border crossings, which is not insignificant. There are four border crossings attended by immigration officers and seventeen "bush paths" between Ghana and Togo, the latter being frequently used on market days. In order to immunize children whose mothers might be bringing them to Ghana during Togo's National Immunization Day exercises, "districts were advised to put teams at all crossing points" (interview, Tamale, 22 May 2009). Nonetheless, some mothers may refuse vaccination or, as traders, may simply not have time (Nichter 1996, 354n28), regardless of whether sufficient health personnel are available during busy market-day crossings.

Communication Networks

Along with the mobility of people and their cattle, there is the mobility of messages, communicated by word of mouth and also by radio. Thus events in Togo or Nigeria may reach the ears of those in Ghana, with consequences for the Polio Eradication Initiative. For example, a school director living in Yendi described the impact that news of the 2003 Kano State polio boycott had on his own family:

> There was a time . . . it wasn't long ago when they heard that in Nigeria, some people received immunization and that some of them fell seriously ill . . . and some thought that they were trying to give them something to control their births in the future. So as a result, they didn't want to do it. I had a personal experience of that . . . [as when] they came to my house, my wife didn't want the children to do it. But when I came back, I explained [it] to her and she told me that this was what she had heard. So I said, "Well, it's not true." So I believe that several people would have declined [for this reason] because even on Radio Tamale, I heard the health education officer at Tamale, he went on the radio and was appealing to people to go for immunization. (Interview, Yendi, 21 May 2009)

Yet it is difficult both to estimate the effect of the 2003–2004 Kano polio vaccination boycott on people in the Northern Region of Ghana and to assess to what extent their suspicions were subsequently allayed. According to the regional manager of the Expanded Programme on Immunisation in Tamale, the Health Department's efforts to dispel this rumor were effective:

> We were lucky that they had a Nigerian WHO doctor from Yobe State [in Northern Nigeria] who was posted here then and was also a Muslim, and he enlightened the people. When the issue was resolved [in Northern Nigeria], he showed people's acceptance of the Polio Eradication Initiative there. (Interview, Tamale, 22 May 2009)

While the news from Northern Nigeria may have raised suspicions about the oral polio vaccine in the Northern Region of Ghana, by 2004 sufficient numbers of parents had been convinced to accept the oral polio vaccine during the four National Immunization Days that year that there were no further outbreaks until 2008.

The transnational movement of certain ethnic groups living in the Northern Region of Ghana and in Northern Nigeria, who travel across permeable national borders in pursuing their work as traders or herders or simply to attend family functions, has contributed to the difficulty of maintaining levels of routine immunization and conducting National Immunization Days. That officials in Ghana managed to keep immunization levels sufficiently high from 2004 to 2007 is evidence of their efforts. That an outbreak nonetheless occurred in the Northern Region in 2008 underscores the challenges they face. One immunization control officer in Yendi observed, with considerable honesty, in response to my question about why these cases occurred in the Northern Region,

> When you look at some of the cases we actually had, in 2003, the case from Yendi [District], the child didn't have good immunization records so you might be tempted to say, well, that some of the mothers don't take the immunization routine. And then in 2008, the [first] case had a good immunization record. Here we are, the child is down with a condition and we don't know how we can assign a clear reason as to why.... But came the second case, it's like 2003, the mother had not taken [her child] for any immunization. So maybe the Northern Region—and I'm not privy to other district cases, whether the immunization records were good or bad—but I'm tempted to generalize that looking at the trend, it seems those children who have not had good immunization status, they are even more [numerous] than children who have good immunization status. So I might draw the conclusion that perhaps here we still have the challenge [to] plan the importance of our services. You see, it may be some of our people are still resistant [to immunization] and that's why in the Northern Region we are still getting these cases related to preventable diseases. I think that is why, in my opinion. (Interview, Yendi, 23 May 2009)

Nonetheless, despite health workers' failure to convince all parents of the benefits of routine immunization for their children, the percentage of Ghanaian children who have been immunized is sufficiently high that there have been relatively few cases of polio paralysis in the past ten years.

* * *

Polio vaccination, introduced mainly through the Expanded Programme on Immunisation, was intensified with the introduction of the Polio Eradication Initiative in 1996 in both Nigeria and Ghana. Despite the uniform protocol of the Initiative, differences in government implementation of the program, as well as in government support for routine immunization, have contributed to significant differences in polio immunization levels and consequently in the number of polio cases. Yet the Northern Region of Ghana is sufficiently similar to Northern Nigeria to suggest that the national boundaries that separate these countries do not always coincide with cultural views.

For example, in both Northern Nigeria and the Northern Region of Ghana, parents who are uncertain about the causes of Shan Inna or *gbalibila fiep-fiep* and about the effects of injections may also be fearful about the safety of the oral polio vaccine. In the Northern Region, the association of diarrhea with oral polio vaccine led some parents to avoid vaccinating their children, while in Northern Nigeria some parents resisted because the vaccine was associated with infertility. In both places, some parents moved with their children to other villages, states, and even countries to avoid vaccination teams. Furthermore, both areas saw political conflict—whether at the local level, as in Yendi District in 1994 and 2002, or at the state or national level, as in Nigeria, which experienced instability in presidential leadership, national strikes, and the politicization of the Nigerian immunization program as well as state boycotts of the polio campaign itself. This conflict led to disruptions in routine immunization and vaccine supplies and contributed to parents' distrust of their government's ability to protect them and their families.

While the three cases of polio in Yendi District in 2003 and 2008 represent three distinctive parental responses to the polio campaign in the Northern Region, the Polio Eradication Initiative has achieved some credibility in the Northern Region of Ghana. This credibility is due, in part, to the provision of primary health care, as evidenced by declines in infant and child mortality (Ghana Statistical Service, Ghana Health Service, and Macro International 2009, 119)[13] and high levels of immunization, and to education campaigns in schools, mosques, and churches. Many, but not all, parents trust that their government is addressing the health problems of their children, and thus are willing to participate in the Polio Eradication Initiative. Thus despite political conflict in the Northern Region, which has impeded health care provision there, regional health officials have persisted in providing basic health care, including routine immunization, to the region's children. If cases of polio of Northern Nigerian origin continue to be reported in the Northern Region, the blame lies not with what is happening in Northern Nigeria but rather with the Northern Region's own program, as one immunization control officer in Yendi explained:

> If that is the case [that the polio cases in Yendi were traced to Northern Nigeria]—and we know that once a child is seroconverted and protected and the virus even comes and is circulating, the child shouldn't contract the disease. And though I've said if Nigeria is importing this thing—they still have the virus—if we reach the level of immunization that is higher, we won't be affected. So while that thing is there anyway, [it will not affect us] if our own people see this routine immunization as something [good] and cooperate really well and our routine immunization levels are really high, I think it will be minimal if it even comes. . . . If our immunization routine is actually 90 percent or beyond that, it will not be possible to transfer the disease. (Interview, Yendi, 23 May 2009)

By comparison, in Northern Nigeria, high levels of infant and child mortality, associated with diseases such as malaria and measles, have contributed to a lack of public trust in the federal government's commitment to addressing primary health care problems, and this lack of trust has undermined routine immunization and eradication efforts there.[14] While the recent inclusion of measles vaccinations and other health incentives in National Immunization Day programs has encouraged many parents to participate, their effect is undermined by the federal failure to improve maternal health care and provide electricity, which is available in all but the remotest areas of Ghana.

Yet, as Aaby has observed, mistakes such as were made in the initial implementation of the polio campaign in Nigeria may at times be made "in the right direction." If some Northern Nigerians' distrust of the focus on polio in the face of their government's inability to provide primary health care and routine immunization has hampered the Polio Eradication Initiative there, it also led to the inception of Immunization Plus Days, community dialogue, and the inclusion of health incentives in 2006. Furthermore, parents' resistance in Northern Nigeria—and in Ghana as well—serves as a reminder that such programs are not easily carried out and may often fail "to confront the contradictions, to see the unplanned, and to question [their] own assumptions" (Aaby 2004, 984). The difficulties of confronting the ethics of eradication, as well as the contradictions and assumptions reflected in the multiple definitions of eradication itself, are the topics of the following chapter.

7. The Ethics of Eradication

I call the night to witness when it covers over, and the day when it shines in all its glory, and Him who created the male and female, that your endeavor is for different ends. Yet he who gives to others and has fear, and affirms goodness, We shall ease the way of fortune for him.

—Qur'an 92:1–7

As William James (1891, 200) has observed, "Various essences of good have thus been found and proposed as bases of the ethical system," although no one "essence" prevails everywhere; there are many ethical frames in the world. While this relativistic position on the constitution of ethical systems sits well with the concept of cultural relativism familiar to anthropologists,[1] it counters the tendency to assume that one's own standards of conduct are the proper, ethical ones. Indeed, the etymology of the word "ethical," which is derived from the Greek word *ethos*, "character, customs, a man's normal state," underscores the local nature of such systems and their grounding in everyday things and practices, as taken-for-granted normalcy. This is not to say that ideas about what constitutes moral behavior—what is good and bad—in different ethical systems are mutually untranslatable and that such systems may never merge. The merging of ethical frames during an era of global campaigns—such as movements to end poverty, to support human rights, and to educate women—is based on a congruence of concerns, even when such general public goods may, nonetheless, be distinctively interpreted.

This analysis of the ethics of eradication—from the perspective of both Northern Nigerian parents and public health officials—is based on the idea that different ethical systems each have their own respective merits and demerits. This belief reflects my own ethical perspective as an anthropologist for whom the analysis of issues from different perspectives is considered preferable, if not always objectively possible. Other professional ethical frames, such as those of public health, may differ. Furthermore, there are different interpretations of ethical practice within the disciplines of anthropology[2] and public health themselves. For example, some public health practitioners may see parental input in public health campaigns as critically important, while others consider the vaccination of children to take precedence over the wishes of individual parents (Bradley 2000b). Alternately, Northern Nigerian parents have their own ethical frames through which they consider the health of their children and their communities. According to one frame, parents are morally responsible for promoting the health and well-being of their children to the best of their ability. When weighing their children's participation in the Polio Eradication Initiative, some parents allude to religious texts and teachings which support their decision to avoid the risks associated with vaccination and with Western medicine more generally.[3] However, in addition to their individual responsibility, parents also expect their government to provide assistance during epidemics and general sanitation programs.

Keeping these different views of individual and state responsibility for child health care in mind, I first consider the ethical concerns of public health practitioners about public health practice, about who should contribute to making decisions about health care priorities, and about who should have access to medical information. This latter point is particularly germane in light of the emergence of circulating vaccine-derived poliovirus, confirmed in 2006 (CDC 2007a; McNeil 2007). I then examine the ethical bases of Northern Nigerian parents' views. Although the World Health Assembly's resolution to eradicate polio was approved by Nigerian government officials, community input into this decision was not sought by Ministry of Health personnel. While Northern Nigerian parents did not expect the sorts of government programs operative in the West, such as the citizens' juries set up in the UK (G. Needham 2000) or the National Vaccine Injury Compensation Program, organized to address parental fears that vaccination caused autism in the U.S. (Edlich et al. 2007), they did expect their government to provide a modicum of free primary health care to its citizens. Some parents decided not to participate in the Polio Eradication Initiative on the grounds that their government was behaving irresponsibly by not addressing their children's lack of primary health care (Renne 2006). Finally, I consider the ethics of eradication as a public health practice. The Gates Foundation's recent call to eradicate malaria and the implicit muting of criticism associated with this decision (McNeil 2008a) underscore the ways that a public health initiative's focus on a single disease raises general ethical concerns about public health priorities, community input, and health care equity. This discussion also calls attention to the ways that international NGOs and foundations decide on and then underwrite public health interventions in low-income countries (Das 1999; Pfeiffer 2004). Evidence from the Northern Nigerian example may lead one to question the ultimate effectiveness of this particular global approach when little or no attempts are made to find a mutually agreeable ground for different ethical frames.

Ethics and Public Health Interventions

Public health ethics is a subset of medical ethics and bioethics, although it is distinctive in its focus on populations, rather than on individuals (Holland 2007). The extensive public health literature regarding ethical concerns discusses health as a public good, community input in public health priorities, and health care as social justice (e.g., Anand, Peter, and Sen 2004; Beauchamp and Steinbock 1999; Bradley and Burls 2000; Holland 2007). One of the fundamental ethical dilemmas for public health practitioners is how to improve the health of communities while preserving individual rights. For example, in order for the transmission of disease to be controlled, a certain percentage of the population must be vaccinated; "herd immunity" is usually considered to require about 80 percent coverage. Individual parents who fail to immunize their children, whether for religious or philosophical reasons or out of fear of the consequences of vaccination (so-called "free riders"), are seen by public health officials as undermining the health of the entire community, and these parents may be subjected to coercive measures. In some countries, such as the U.S., immunization levels of more than 90 percent have been obtained through an improved system of vaccine delivery, including free vaccines for children of low-income families, as well as laws requiring children to be vaccinated before entering primary school (Colgrove 2006, 248). In other countries, such as the UK, strong primary health care programs encourage parents' voluntary immunization of their children through frequent mailings and home visits (Bradley 2000b; Holland 2007). Such programs also rely on extensive surveillance of vital statistics, medical records, and immunization counts, and this surveillance may raise ethical concerns about privacy and data accuracy.

Public health ethics are concerned with health care equity, particularly in situations where resources are limited (Bradley 2000a). Health officials consider immunization, which prevents disease, "one of the most cost-effective public health interventions available" (Brenzel et al. 2006, 389). They may also consider mass immunization the most equitable strategy, since all children, regardless of their socioeconomic backgrounds, may obtain vaccinations during public health campaigns at little or no cost (Bonu, Rani, and Baker 2003). Eradication initiatives which go to great lengths to immunize children living in remote and impoverished areas have been so described by the former head of the Carter Center, Dr. William Foege, who noted that "the bottom line is that eradication attacks inequities and provides the ultimate social justice" (Hull and Aylward 2001, 4383).

Ideally, public health activities, such as mass immunization campaigns, health education and promotion, and disease surveillance programs, are carried out to benefit entire populations, while still respecting the rights of individuals and communities. However, in practice, time and funding constraints have sometimes led to unethical public health practices, as when strong coercive measures were used during the final years of the smallpox eradication campaign in South Asia, e.g., entering private homes and forcibly vaccinating occupants (Greenough 1995), or when quarantine measures were used in an effort to control the spread of HIV-AIDS (Castro and Singer 2004).

The differential treatment of populations in low-income and high-income countries also raises questions concerning public health ethics and the ways in which they are conceptualized and discussed. While the ethics of public health programs in high-income countries may be couched in terms of human rights, in low-income countries they may be framed in terms of basic services, without an ethical component. Thus "diseases of the affluent"—such as HIV-AIDS—attract extensive ethical discussion, while long-standing "diseases of the poor"—such as measles or cholera, which have been essentially eliminated in the West—are rarely considered from an ethical perspective (Das 1999, 101). This ethical prioritizing of some infectious diseases, and not others, reflects anxieties about globalization, about keeping the movements of people and disease under control through immigration restrictions and immunization programs. To some extent, decisions made by global institutional officials and NGOs with the authority and funds to determine public health priorities reflect the relative positions of those who see themselves as being jeopardized and those who are seen as contributing to these global flows of infection.

The particular ethical dilemma of who should decide public health priorities was raised by Taylor, Cutts, and Taylor (1997) with respect to the Polio Eradication Initiative. Health officials' focus on eradicating polio, by distributing oral polio vaccine and establishing a protocol for surveillance of acute flaccid paralysis and testing of fecal samples, tended to override other primary health care measures (Kimman and Boot 2006). Yet it was precisely these measures which would have assuaged the ethical concerns of Northern Nigerian parents.

The Ethical Frames of Northern Nigerian Parents

Parents' expectation that the Nigerian government would provide basic primary health care services derives, in part, from provision of public health services by the colonial government (Schram 1971), which was continued during the Independence era. In Northern Nigeria, the state's obligations to its tax-paying citizens paralleled earlier political relationships between emirs and their subjects. In the Zaria Emirate, for example, tribute (during the precolonial period) and taxes (under the colonial regime) were paid to the emir, with the expectation that he and his officers would look after commoners' interests, just as the family head (*mai gida*) has a moral responsibility to protect his family, while family members in turn respect his authority.

However, as was discussed in chapter 3, the vagaries of primary health care provision in Nigeria have reflected the country's political instability—the period from 1985 to 2008 witnessed seven different heads of state. The shift from a primary health care program run by the federal government to one run by local governments and supported by user fees (in accordance with World Bank and IMF requirements), the privatization of health care, and the installation of a military president with little concern for public health all contributed to a decline in basic health services during the 1990s. While people continued to believe that basic health services were the responsibility of the government, they adapted to government lapses by seeking private health care when necessary—which, for the very poor, meant seeking diagnoses and treatments from chemist shops and traditional healers, whose services they could afford (Alubo 1990). The federal government's failure to provide basic health care undermined the reciprocity of the state-citizen relationship. Thus, when the federal government promoted the Polio Eradication Initiative, some parents questioned the focus on polio rather than primary health care provision and felt little obligation to comply.

Fractures in this relationship were evident when, in 2005, the Toro Local Government Council in Bauchi State announced that "any parent that prevents his or her child from being immunized stands the risk of a jail term" (Hallah 2005). And in March 2008, the traditional ruler of Dikwa in Borno State instructed district and village heads to report the names of parents who had not allowed their children to be vaccinated (N. Musa 2008). While such decrees might seem ethical, considering that in 2008 Northern Nigeria had the largest number of confirmed wild poliovirus cases in the world, their ethics may also be questioned, since vaccines and basic primary health care are often not available. Such dilemmas pit "one right against another right" (Das 1999, 113). In response to these coercive measures, parents relied on an arsenal of "weapons of the weak," which included hiding children or moving them to areas where no such rulings were enacted. Some even "chased away the vaccinators who had braced the cold to immunize the children" (Rabiu 2008a).

Northern Nigerian parents also argue that a focus on polio eradication impedes the equitable distribution of health services. These questions were raised in a discussion described by one Ahmadu Bello University professor:

> Somebody asked me this question . . . and he's a very enlightened person . . . , "Professor, do you believe in these causes we are talking about, child survival strategy and programs?" . . . I said, "Absolutely!" He said, "You're talking about equity, equity." I said, "Yes, I believe in equity." And he said, "All right. You must be misled by these Western blocs, Western powers. But in your own honest opinion, Professor, tell me, what kills most children here—is it malaria or polio?" I said, "Yes, it's malaria. Malaria kills immediately. But that polio may not kill but have a permanent damage, would affect the economic output of people. . . ." He said, "No"; as far as he's concerned, if I agree malaria is the problem, why don't they concentrate on malaria? "And they are emphasizing polio. Is that your equity?" (Interview, Zaria, 20 July 2005)

This man understood equity in a somewhat different way from those supporting eradication programs, who see universal polio vaccination as a form of equitable health care and as the "ultimate social justice." For him, the emphasis on polio, rather than on the more lethal childhood disease of malaria, was an inequitable focus on a relatively small number of children and an inequitable distribution of health resources.

Health care equity is also related to questions about public health priorities and who should have a voice in setting them. In Northern Nigeria, the ethics of the public health mandate to focus on community, rather than individual, health are complicated in the case of the Polio Eradication Initiative by people's belief that the Initiative was driven by Western interests, not their own. Furthermore, many Northern Nigerian parents believe that they should have more authority over their children's health than the state, particularly when they do not see the federal government upholding its health care responsibilities. This belief does not mean that they cannot be convinced to immunize their children—immunization days sponsored by local rulers such as the Emir of Zaria, or by community leaders such as the man known as "7-Up" in Zaria City, have persuaded many parents to permit health workers to vaccinate their children for polio and other childhood diseases. However, parents should make these decisions in accordance with their own beliefs, as one young mother whose child was immunized without her consent at a primary school in Zaria City explained:

> Children are born with natural immunity from God. People will only improve the one God has given by giving injections. For example, children will eat so many things, but when they are small, they will eat what they are given by their parents, and their parents will try to give them clean and good food and they will have good health. But when they are older, they will eat many things and will be more in need of injections.
>
> Natural immunity is the real immunization. The other immunization is not important because I never had it. If God wishes, the one who had immunization will be sick but the one who didn't have immunization will be in good health. But immunization can protect a person if the person believes in it and [also believes] that it is only God who will protect them. . . .
>
> Islam believes in immunization because God said, "Wake up and I will help you." It's not that God says it is not good, it is just that people don't want it . . . that's why they don't take immunization. And there are some who don't take Western medicine, they only take traditional medicine. (Interview, Zaria City, 24 July 2007)

Coercive measures such as giving children vaccine without parental consent may be effective in the short term, but they may foster resentment which may undermine future efforts to implement routine immunization (Greenough 1995, 643). While parents in the U.S. are legally required to vaccinate their children prior to their entering school—which some see as a coercive measure—they may petition to have their children exempted from vaccination on religious or philosophical grounds (Colgrove 2006, 180). Nigerian parents do not have this option, although in 2008 parents of school children in Zaria were allowed to send letters to school principals requesting that their children not be immunized (personal communication, May 2009). Yet because of their experience of mandatory colonial health measures, some older Northern Nigerians might not expect to have options like those available to U.S. parents; this double standard in the ethics of international public health interventions has a historical basis. Indeed, from the perspective of Northern Nigerian parents, it was a lack of an appropriate ethical approach to informed consent that marred the trial of the antibiotic Trovan in Kano, Nigeria, in 1996, which has also had consequences for the acceptance of the Polio Eradication Initiative there.

The Pfizer Trovan Drug Trial

In 1996, an epidemic of cerebrospinal meningitis occurred in Northern Nigeria, with Kano State being particularly hard hit (WHO 1996b). There were more than 20,982 cases of cerebrospinal meningitis that year, with 3,634 deaths from the disease (WHO 1996a). Prior to the epidemic's outbreak in early January, the Nigerian government had not provided sufficient meningitis vaccine, nor were sufficient drug treatments available after it began (Ejembi, Renne, and Adamu 1998). Officials with the pharmaceutical corporation Pfizer, Inc., having learned about this situation from an Internet site (Lewin 2001), organized a trial of the antibiotic Trovan (trovafloxacin) at a hospital in Kano. Although Trovan been used as an antibiotic for adults in the U.S., its association with liver damage and death led to its use being severely restricted, and it was banned in Europe. It had never been approved for use in children (Stephens 2006).

During the trial, the oral form of Trovan was given to approximately one hundred children brought to the Infectious Disease Hospital in Kano for treatment of cerebrospinal meningitis; another hundred children were given the antibiotic Cephtriaxone, the standard treatment, as a control, although Cephtriaxone was given at a lower than recommended dosage (Lenzer 2007).[4] Of the children involved in the study, eleven subsequently died—five who had been given Trovan, six who had been given Cephtriaxone. Although it was not publicized at the time, news of the trial became widespread in Nigeria after the *Washington Post* published a story on it in 2000 (Stephens 2000). Consequently, a blue-ribbon panel held a hearing in Kano in January 2001 and a lawsuit was filed by families of some of the affected children in a New York district court in 2002. In the suit, the families claimed that Pfizer conducted a clinical drug trial on foreign citizens without their consent (Obadare 2005; Olusanya 2004; Petryna 2005). This case was dismissed on the grounds that it was out of the court's jurisdiction (*Abdullahi vs. Pfizer, Inc.* 2005), and efforts were made to reopen the trial in Nigeria. However, the trial was delayed until 2006, when the publication of another *Washington Post* article on the 2001 Trovan hearing reinvigorated efforts to secure restitution.[5] Subsequently, in June 2007, the Nigerian federal government and the Kano State government filed a criminal suit against Pfizer and eight other defendants, charging that they had given an untested drug to children without obtaining adequate informed consent (Suleiman 2007, 49). The case was adjourned until October 2007 (Rabiu 2007, 2), and a suit brought by the Kano State government was reopened in March 2008. After considerable maneuvering, which involved Kano State government officials and two former heads of state, President Yakubu Gowon and President Jimmy Carter, the U.S. district court's dismissal of the parents' case was overturned (Lenzer 2009). In March 2009, Pfizer and Kano State officials, along with representatives of the children's families, met to confirm an out-of-court settlement for US$75 million (Abdullah 2009a, 2009b; Washington Post 2009).

The 1996 Trovan drug trial raises a number of questions about biomedical research in low-income countries where economic factors, including payments to local medical personnel, may override ethical concerns. The chief issue on which the lawsuits rested, the informed consent of the parents, also raises the question of whether drug trials should be conducted during disease epidemics when parents—frantic to find treatment for their desperately ill children—may not fully understand the potential consequences of giving untested drugs to their children. The controversy also had consequences for future health interventions. The Trovan drug trial and the lawsuits which followed are still remembered by people in Northern Nigeria, who refer to them as "Pfizer," and people's fears about Trovan have reinforced more general suspicions of Western pharmaceutical companies and

Western biomedicine, as well as of polio immunization (Achebe 2004; Jegede 2007; Obadare 2005). The distrust raised by the Trovan drug trial and the Nigerian government's role in it has led some Northern Nigerians to question their government's ability to protect them from health projects initiated by outsiders, including the Polio Eradication Initiative (Aliyu 2008).

Public Disclosure and Circulating Vaccine-Derived Poliovirus

Ethical questions about the conduct of the Polio Eradication Initiative acquired another dimension with the appearance of cases of vaccine-derived poliovirus, which began in July 2005 (CDC 2007a, 2007b). Early signs of a problem appeared in 2003, when genetic sequencing of two polio case samples revealed slight genetic deviations from the oral polio vaccine (Adu et al. 2003). In 2005, the first case of circulating vaccine-derived poliovirus was identified in Gombe State in Northern Nigeria (Adu et al. 2007), although the extent of the outbreak was not known until 2006, when a cluster of type 2 poliovirus samples from Northern Nigeria were sent to the Centers for Disease Control, Atlanta. As type 2 wild poliovirus had been eradicated globally since 1999, a lab technician suspected that these might be vaccine-derived strains which had mutated from trivalent oral polio vaccine given in 2004 (Roberts 2007b). This suspicion was confirmed by a closer analysis of these samples, which showed a greater than 1 percent nucleotide sequence deviation from the Sabin oral polio vaccine (CDC 2007a; CDC 2007b, 966; WHO 2007d).[6] After the initial case in 2005, 21 cases of vaccine-derived poliovirus were confirmed to have occurred in 2006, 68 cases in 2007, 62 cases in 2008, and 103 cases in the first six months of 2009 (CDC 2009a).

The outbreak of vaccine-derived poliovirus in Northern Nigeria presented a difficult ethical dilemma for Ministry of Health, WHO, and CDC officials. In order to stop it from spreading, they needed to vaccinate as many children as possible with trivalent oral polio vaccine. They feared that if they made the news of the vaccine-derived poliovirus outbreak public, it could contribute to rumors about the dangers of oral polio vaccine, with parents then refusing to allow their children to be immunized (Roberts 2007b). They therefore decided to continue with the immunization campaign in 2006 and 2007, without announcing the presence of vaccine-derived poliovirus. However, after an international meeting on polio held at the National Institutes of Health in Bethesda, Maryland, in early September 2007, at which the significant reduction in wild poliovirus cases as of August 2007 and the outbreak of vaccine-derived poliovirus were discussed, news of the outbreak was publicly released.[7] Nonetheless, some government officials continued to be uneasy and tried to prevent the public from hearing about the outbreak (Walker 2007a).

Yet news of vaccine-derived poliovirus infections does not seem to have spread, and predictions of new rumors apparently have not proven correct. Although stories about the outbreak appeared in several Nigerian newspapers (e.g., *Punch, Daily Trust*) and on the BBC website (A. Last 2007; Walker 2007b), many people in Zaria, at least, had not heard about vaccine-derived poliovirus. For example, the head of a polio vaccination team in one local government did not know about it, nor did a pediatrician associated with Ahmadu Bello University

Teaching Hospital.[8] The general public associates polio with paralysis, and the complicated process by which the attenuated poliovirus used in oral polio vaccine may mutate into a dangerous form—a process which may take many months or even years—may be difficult to imagine or understand. It is also possible that a detailed knowledge of the process whereby attenuated poliovirus reverts to a virulent form may simply not be considered worth knowing about (Last 1981). The fact that fully immunized children do not get polio directly from oral polio vaccine after being vaccinated and that it can protect them from both wild poliovirus and vaccine-derived poliovirus also makes it less likely that news of circulating vaccine-derived poliovirus will undermine polio immunization efforts.

Regardless of how the vaccine-derived poliovirus outbreak was viewed by Northern Nigerian parents, the fact that news of it was withheld is ethically problematic on several grounds. These grounds include public access to health information (and, implicitly, informed consent), respect for the knowledge of community members, and the honest presentation of scientific research. Regarding the first issue, the decision to withhold the news in 2006, for fear of rumors and anti-vaccination sentiment, made sense in that it was precisely further immunization that was necessary in order to limit the spread of circulating vaccine-derived poliovirus. Yet if communication of health information is one of the ethical mandates of public health practice, the news should have been made public as it became known. By not doing so, those involved with the Polio Eradication Initiative undermined their portrayal of the campaign as a moral and responsible effort to prevent children's being paralyzed by poliomyelitis, without a hidden agenda. Furthermore, the decision not to release this information suggested a lack of respect for the intelligence not only of residents of Northern Nigerian communities but also of the general international public. One WHO polio program official was quoted as saying that the failure to release information on vaccine-derived poliovirus until August 2007 "was an oversight on our part" rather than an intentional decision to suppress this information (McNeil 2007). Another said "that because the organization considered the outbreak to be a problem for scientists and not something that would change global vaccination practices, they thought it was unnecessary to immediately share [this information] publicly" (Cheng 2007). Yet the misrepresentation of numerical data on the WHO website not only undermines the credibility of the Polio Eradication Initiative figures, but also reinforces questions about the validity of data on routine immunization presented by WHO elsewhere (Das 1999; Hardon and Blume 2005, 347).[9]

However, not all Polio Eradication Initiative and public health workers agreed with the decision to withhold information about cases of circulating vaccine-derived poliovirus in Nigeria. Some feared that the consequences of not releasing the information in a timely fashion would be worse than those of doing so. Others hoped that more could be learned about the dynamics of vaccine-derived polio-viruses (Roberts 2007b). The ethical dilemma of whether and when to publicize the outbreak of vaccine-derived poliovirus in Northern Nigeria underscores the difficulties and the sometimes unexpected consequences of conducting an eradication campaign. Yet eradication initiatives have particular characteristics that tend to incline those involved toward making decisions in one way and not in others.

The Meaning of Eradication

The term "eradication" (from the Latin *eradicare,* "to uproot") is something of an "odd-job" word (R. Needham 1971, 5) that has taken on so many different meanings in the popular vernacular that its meaning in the context of public health has been blurred. Indeed, public health practitioners have not agreed upon its definition (Dowdle 1998; Goodman et al. 1998; Miller, Barrett, and Henderson 2006, 1164; Yekutiel 1980). While the etymology of the word makes it appear to be a straightforward binary—something is uprooted or it is not—it has several interpretations in the public health context. For some, it means the complete extinction of a particular disease pathogen. For others, it means the continued lack of transmission of such a pathogen, which may be specified for a particular place and time frame. Some definitions allow the time frame to vary but insist that eradication must be global, not regional. Yekutiel proposed a definition which provides a useful basis for comparison: "The purposeful reduction of specific disease prevalence to the point of continued absence of transmission within a specified area by means of a time-limited campaign." For him, the time period should be approximately eight years and consist of four phases: a preparatory phase (one year); an "attack" phase (one to two years), when interventions such as mass immunization take place; a consolidation phase (two to three years), consisting of a period of surveillance beginning only after disease transmission has been interrupted or the disease exists at very low levels and no further measures are necessary to prevent its resurgence; and a maintenance phase (three years; what some refer to as post-eradication), during which general health services and lab testing facilities are provided (Yekutiel 1980, 5–6, 25–27).[10]

More recently, Miller, Barrett, and Henderson have dropped the idea of regional eradication. For them, disease eradication has three characteristics: "it is global"; it is characterized by "the certified total absence of human cases, the absence of a reservoir for the organism in nature, and absolute containment of any infectious source"; and "it is binary . . . a disease is certified as either eradicated or not" (Miller, Barrett, and Henderson 2006, 1164).[11] While they do not specify an overall time frame, they expect that the period after transmission has been interrupted—what Yekutiel refers to as the consolidation phase—would consist of a particular period of time (three years in the case of smallpox eradication). During this time there would be few, if any, cases of the disease. At the end of this period there would be a "total absence of human cases," and eradication of the disease would be certified. Indeed, it is important to specify a time frame in defining eradication:

> There is an essential difference between the concepts of eradication and control. Once eradication is achieved the infection is gone forever, and the *costly burden of recurring control measures may be dropped.* If procedures need to be continued to

prevent return of the infection, then the state is one of control and not eradication. (Cockburn 1963, 134, italics in original)

The continually changing time frame of the Polio Eradication Initiative has contributed to the considerable confusion about what the word "eradication" means. In order to reduce the sense that the campaign is proceeding endlessly, some use the term to mean an interruption in the transmission of the disease organism. According to this definition, the period of time prior to certification is then referred to as the "post-eradication" period (see Knobler, Lederberg, and Pray 2002). However, since "procedures need to be continued to prevent the return of the infection," namely continued widespread vaccination with either inactivated polio vaccine or attenuated oral polio vaccine, others have questioned this usage. Not only is continued use of oral polio vaccine required, but there remains the possibility of vaccine-derived poliovirus outbreaks. "The termination of wild virus transmission does not guarantee eradication of poliomyelitis disease, considering that OPV viruses are transmissible and are known to revert back to wild-type phenotype" (Fine and Griffiths 2007, 1321). Indeed, the appearance of circulating vaccine-derived poliovirus has led some to revise the definition of polio eradication specifically to include the "total absence of human cases" caused by both wild and vaccine-derived poliovirus (Ehrenfeld et al. 2008, 1385). According to this definition, attenuated oral polio vaccine must have been replaced by inactivated polio vaccine and "a total absence of human cases" must have existed for at least three years before the eradication of polio can be certified. "By definition, in a post-eradication scenario, there will be no further need for any strategy against either poliomyelitis or poliovirus. In short, there is no such thing as a 'post-eradication immunization policy'" (Razum et al. 2004, 2191). Unless, that is, a new definition of eradication can be mutually agreed upon.

In Nigeria, the word "eradication" has been used by health officials to mean both "a total absence of human cases" and "the interruption of transmission." For example, in April 2008, the governor of Kano State, Ibrahim Shekarau, announced that "his administration was determined to help in total eradication of the disease from the country" (Karofi 2008a).[12] The governor also situated his actions within a larger rhetoric of development, speaking of polio eradication as part of "the achievement of an effective health care delivery in the state." Similarly, in 2005, former president Obasanjo described his administration's support for the Polio Eradication Initiative as part of the agenda of the Millennium Development Goals, formulated by the UN and WHO:

Polio, the president observed, is on the brink of eradication world wide after small pox and that efforts are being made to stop transmission of the wild polio virus by the end of this year as his administration is fully committed to the survival and improvement of health of children as emphasized in the National Economic Empowerment Development Strategy (NEEDS) and the Millenium Development Goals. (Oroye 2005)

While the practical consequences of such programmatic lists of ideal development goals and strategies have been questioned, the eradication of polio, in the sense in which Razum et al. (2004) define it, would be beneficial for Nigeria in that it would end polio vaccination costs. Furthermore, these political leaders emphasize that eradicating polio would improve Nigeria's reputation in the community of nations. Nigeria is often cited as one of the last four countries in the world to harbor wild poliovirus, which, like the presence of beggars (as discussed in chapter 5), is an embarrassment for its leaders.[13]

National leaders and health officials also discuss polio eradication in terms of children's health, which is the primary concern voiced by community health workers and parents. For example, one ward focal officer working for the Zaria Local Government Department of Health noted that during Immunization Plus Days his team would go to areas where polio immunization coverage was low "in order to tell them of the importance of immunizing their children" (interview, Zaria, 2 August 2007). One mother also focused on the benefits of the polio vaccine to children's health: "Since they said they want to do away with the disease, in order to have good health, there is no fault in it, it has no effect. Because one likes everyone to have good health, so I am supporting the program" (interview, Zaria, 6 July 2005). Her reference to eradication ("do[ing] away with the disease") may have been the result of being told of the importance of eradication by immunization team mobilizers. One young woman vaccinator explained, "Like me, if I'm going to be the mobilizer, sometimes what I used to tell them [was] we are all Muslims and we are sisters. You know we will not cheat you in this vaccine. If we know it is not good, we will not come and ask you to take it, as we are all Muslims and we are sisters in Islam. And as smallpox [*ciwon 'yar rani*] was eradicated, we want to eradicate [*kawar*, remove] polio too" (interview, Zaria, 31 August 2005).

People may also have learned about eradication from television and radio spots promoting the Polio Eradication Initiative. In these media promotions, as well as on bags, caps, and T-shirts, the polio eradication campaign is promoted by the soccer-based slogan, "Kick Polio Out of Africa." The growth of media publicity for eradication campaigns such as the Polio Eradication Initiative reflects twentieth-century developments in the recording and television industries, as well as changes in advertisement and marketing strategies from print media to radio and television. These developments, along with improvements in vaccines, antibiotics, and technologies for vaccine delivery and for the elimination of disease vectors (such as DDT spraying for mosquitos), have enabled public health officials to imagine new ways in which such programs can be run.

In the expectation that advances in medical science and technology could make it possible to eradicate diseases, programs focusing on malaria (in 1955), yaws (in 1955), and smallpox (in 1967) were begun with much confidence. However, as a result of ecological factors (such as DDT-resistant mosquitos and DDT-related environmental hazards), biological factors (such as subclinical cases of yaws), and operational factors (such as the difficulty of surveillance), only the smallpox program met the criteria of eradication set out by Miller, Barrett, and

Henderson. But despite these setbacks, there is something about the concept of eradication that leads donors and public health personnel alike to become seduced by the challenge to end, once and for all, the transmission of a particular infectious disease (Henderson 1998). Eradication efforts are attractive not just for humanitarian and economic reasons, but also because of their narrow focus and their uniform protocol, decided upon by a relatively small group of individuals with significant resources and authority. One might say that this quality of eradication infects those involved in eradication efforts who, in their single-mindedness of purpose, often do not look kindly on different or critical points of view. Such single-mindedness tends to discourage questions about possible impediments to the effort's success and tends to suppress opposition as an illegitimate obstruction. This dynamic is suggested by a recent *New York Times* story about the Gates Foundation's recent decision to pursue the eradication of malaria:

> One week after the Gates announcement, the head of an organization financed by the foundation joked in front of a small audience that eradication was "the new marching order."
>
> "Go along with it if you want to get funded," he said, adding that it was viable only if linked "to a date like 2050, or far enough in the future so that none of us can be held accountable."
>
> Asked about that afterward, he asked that he not be quoted. In subsequent forums, he stopped joking and repeatedly said eradication was his organization's goal. (McNeil 2008a)

This way of thinking, which does not bridge opposition, also counters some of the ethical concerns about community input, health priorities, and access to information raised by public health practitioners discussed above. It may affect the implementation of eradication campaigns, both directly, through recourse to coercive vaccination practices (Andrews 2006; Greenough 1995), and indirectly, through the suppression of negative information and through the perpetuation of structural inequalities (Farmer 1999). In the latter case, international donors and medical and public health specialists organizing and funding eradication initiatives determine global health priorities and initiatives; local communities do not (Pfeiffer 2004).

The Ethics of Eradication

As is the case with public health initiatives more generally, the ethics of eradication can be interpreted in several ways. One might argue that coercive measures, like those used in smallpox eradication campaigns, may be warranted in light of the benefits of eradicating such diseases. One might also argue that eradication initiatives which rely on coercive immunization practices, either directly or indirectly, are not only unethical but also counterproductive. As Greenough has noted, the success of the South Asian smallpox eradication campaign in the early 1970s "demonstrated the technical feasibility of disease eradication as a significant public health strategy." Yet it is not only the distinctive organizational, financial and epidemiological methods that have been transmitted forward from the SEP [Smallpox Eradication Program]; so have the aggressive attitudes and values that came to underpin it in its most successful moments during the mid-1970s. These attitudes and values, it might be argued, served the SEP well in the context of a disease *eradication campaign,* but they make a bad fit with the requirements of a disease *control programme.* Few communicable diseases, in fact, are suitable for eradication, and in most cases the best that can be hoped for is to control a disease's spread. . . . In short, unwonted aggressiveness in delivering immunization is unsuited to building sustainable vaccination programs. (Greenough 1995, 643)

An aggressive focus on the eradication of a single disease can foster distrust of immunization, and, as Greenough observed, "Once public opinion turns against state-enforced measures, the task of the health workers become much more difficult." Taking account of the ethical frameworks of others is something inherently antithetical to the singular focus of eradication efforts. Yet a failure to do so makes health workers' tasks more difficult. As a result of increased resistance, their task may be more time-consuming and ultimately more expensive.

Yet the ideological shift in the 1990s—from broad-based health projects such as the Expanded Programme on Immunisation to disease eradication programs and technological innovations such as the genetic sequencing of enteroviruses utilized by the Polio Eradication Initiative—was propelled largely by economic considerations (Hardon and Blume 2005, 348). If such projects proceed according to plan, they may indeed be more cost-effective than open-ended disease control interventions (Barrett 2004; Thompson and Tebbens 2007). However, as Yekutiel (1980, 21) has cautioned, "the heavy capital investment will only pay off if eradication is achieved reasonably well within the planned period of time. . . . [If not,] there is considerable risk of losing not only the 'pay off' but the capital as well."[14] It remains to be seen what the ultimate costs of the Polio Eradication Initiative may be. This uncertainty exists, in part, because it is not known when wild poliovirus transmission will cease and to what extent outbreaks of vaccine-derived poliovirus may re-emerge in low-income countries where oral polio vaccine continues to be used.[15] If wild poliovirus transmission is stopped in Nigeria, the post-transmission, precertification period will require continued vaccination with either attenuated oral polio vaccine or inactivated polio vaccine, as well as an extensive surveillance program to monitor whether new cases of polio emerge, which includes significant costs for labs, testing, and local oversight. Thus, while international agencies and donors may view focused interventions such as the Polio Eradication Initiative as the most appropriate means of promoting health care equity and social justice, the differences in countries' ability to provide basic health services—along with the expenses and infrastructure required by long-term eradication efforts—undermine this equity.

Ethical Governance and Eradication

When the Polio Eradication Initiative was launched in 1988, the strengthening of primary health care and routine immunization was one of its objectives.

That this has not happened in Nigeria raises the question whether the different ethical frames—that of international public health practitioners and foundations supporting eradication initiatives as equitable and economical social justice, and that of Northern Nigerian parents who see primary health care programs as the responsibility of government and as a basic human right—can be brought together. Clearly, in West African countries such as Ghana and The Gambia, which have well-organized primary health care infrastructures and health care delivery systems, eradication campaigns can successfully coexist with routine immunization programs (Leach and Fairhead 2007).[16] In Nigeria, however, many years of government neglect of primary health care and of public infrastructure more generally have undermined public health officials' ability to implement an eradication campaign such as the Polio Eradication Initiative. Indeed, public discontent with Nigerian political leaders' apparent disregard for the living conditions of the majority of Nigerians has been expressed in a range of popular culture venues, including newspapers and magazines, videos, poems, and songs, some of which make references to polio in various ways. In the Hausa song "Ba mu yarda tazarce ba" (We Don't Agree That You Continue On, i.e., for a third term) that became popular in 2006, Haruna Aliyu Ninji sings of the ways that President Olusegun Obasanjo (1999–2007), his administration, and his unethical political allies impoverished the country, turning Nigeria into a disabled lame person (*gurgu*), much as the poliovirus does to individuals:

> Also, we are talking about natural resources, the wealth of the country. He went all over the world to get people to invest in Nigeria. But the people didn't come, and the economy of the country became like a lame person [*gurgu*]. He only gathered the money for himself and left the country in poverty. (Ninji 2006)[17]

*　　*　　*

In Northern Nigeria, this view of the former president, during whose tenure polio eradication efforts were intensified, cannot be separated from the operation of the Polio Eradication Initiative itself. His support for the former head of the National Programme on Immunization, Dr. Dere Awosika—a close friend of his late wife who was viewed as both authoritarian and financially suspect—reinforced people's perception that Obasanjo's support of the Polio Eradication Initiative was yet another way to enrich himself and his relations.[18] Obasanjo was ultimately unsuccessful in continuing on (*tazarce*) for a third term (*New York Times* 2006). Furthermore, his hand-picked successor, President Umaru Yar'Adua, has distanced himself from Obasanjo's excesses, although a relation of Obasanjo continued to head the National Primary Health Care Development Agency until October 2008. Whether Yar'Adua is able to counter the distrust surrounding the Polio Eradication Initiative will depend to a large extent on whether he can revitalize the provision of primary health care in Northern Nigeria and can address basic infrastructural problems such as lack of electricity, water, and sanitation, which Nigerians see the government as ethically responsible for providing to its citizens.

In Nigeria, with its large and diverse population and its fragile primary health care system, government and NGO health workers have been under tremendous pressure to distribute vaccines, transport and test stool samples, reduce polio case counts, raise funds, and calm suspicions of the Polio Eradication Initiative. The enormity of these tasks has led to a focus on polio alone, while primary health care and routine immunization have languished in many Northern Nigerian states. Immunization Plus Days, a broad-based public health initiative introduced in mid-2006, provided antimalaria drugs, bednets, deworming medication, and soap along with routine immunizations, contributing to a significant decline in confirmed cases of wild poliovirus, from 1,122 cases in 2006 to 285 cases in 2007 (WHO 2009). However, leadership problems and funding restraints (bednets were no longer offered after 2007) have hampered these efforts, and the number of cases increased in 2008. Nonetheless, by moving away from a focus on polio to a program that included polio immunization along with other vaccines and medicines, and with the strong support of Muslim leaders, public health officials addressed Northern Nigerian parents' expectations of government responsibility for providing a modicum of basic primary health care for its citizens. Consequently, the number of cases has declined again in 2009 (see table 1.1).

Much of the underlying argument over polio eradication in Nigeria centered on whose ethical framework mattered most. Eventually, it became evident that what was needed was a way of bringing these ethical frameworks—one which saw eradication as an efficient and equitable global good, and one which saw primary health care as a basic right of Nigerian citizens—together. As one Nigerian professor deeply involved in the Polio Eradication Initiative in Nigeria observed, medical and public health personnel need to respect the knowledge and expectations of Nigerian parents:

> I think we tend to underestimate the intelligence of the people with whom we have been dealing. I went to a village and people asked me, "Did your father get [his children] vaccinated?" There are ways to explain this. So I said, "Yes, my father has four [living] children—but he had twenty children, [sixteen of whom] wouldn't have died, most likely, if they had been immunized." (Interview, Lagos, 21 February 2008)

Indeed, several university professors viewed the early years of the Polio Eradication Initiative as a missed opportunity, saying that improvements in primary health care at that time, including the reliable provision of routine immunization without charge, would have brought more parents into hospitals and clinics, where their concerns about vaccination might have been better addressed. According to one, such programs must be continued in order for the polio campaign ultimately to succeed:

> What I would advocate, most of the states that have been clear [of polio]—they need vigilance and there has to be political will. . . . The progress they have made so far has been because of routine immunization, not because of mass immunization for polio. (Interview, Ibadan, 22 February 2008)

In Northern Nigeria, resistance to programs such as the Polio Eradication Initiative reflects the need to take different ethical frameworks of health care into account when considering global public health programs, and to find spaces where these frameworks coincide. The epilogue that follows considers this approach in relation to the possible futures for the Polio Eradication Initiative in Northern Nigeria.

Epilogue

Government magic,
Water dey go, water dey come,
Government magic,
Dem dey turn electric to candle.

—Fela Anikulapo-Kuti, "Unknown Soldier"

It is entirely possible that the nonimmunized children come from families that are the most vulnerable to economic and political exigencies in the first instance and are fighting for survival . . . [in] the kind of local context in which the zeal for a government program such as immunization may be met with relative apathy in comparison to the other needs to ensure the survival of a child.

—Das, "Public good, ethics, and everyday life"

In 1967, the CDC launched a nationwide immunization campaign to eradicate measles in the U.S. After an initial sharp decline in cases of measles the following year, their number more than doubled in 1970, and by 1971 it had tripled. Public health officials acknowledged that the measles eradication initiative was foundering. As one infectious disease specialist noted, part of the problem was that measles was not perceived as a major health threat: "The measles immunization program is *for* the people, but it is done *to* the people, not *with* the people, and certainly not as a response to a felt need *of* the people" (Colgrove 2006, 167, 170). In the U.S., it was polio, not measles, that was seen as a major health problem.

The reverse is the case in Northern Nigeria. It is measles, not polio, that parents consider a major health problem (Schimmer and Ihekweazu 2006). In Zaria City alone, measles was reported to have led to the deaths of approximately two hundred children in the fall of 2007 (Babadoko 2007b). Many Northern Nigerian parents are anxious to vaccinate their children against this disease and others, such as cerebrospinal meningitis, which they see as major threats to their children's health,[1] although problems of access to clinics, availability of vaccines, and injectible vaccines poorly administered by health workers have hindered their efforts to immunize their children.

The U.S. measles eradication campaign and the Northern Nigerian Polio Eradication Initiative share another similarity. In both instances, routine immunization provision was (or is) inadequate. In the U.S., at the time of initial measles eradication efforts, primary health clinics had short hours or were not conveniently located, and vaccines were expensive, making it particularly difficult for low-income parents to immunize their children. In Northern Nigeria, primary health care centers are sometimes difficult to get to and transportation may be costly, especially for those living in rural areas. More importantly, vaccines have not been reliably available (FBA Health Systems Analysts 2005), discouraging those who travel long distances to reach a clinic and then are unable to have their children immunized from trying again.

While Nigerian public health and government officials attempted to address these problems through the implementation of Immunization Plus Days in 2006 and through discussions with community and religious leaders, changes in the National Programme on Immunization leadership and organization also contributed to improved levels of immunization. Consequently, confirmed cases of wild poliovirus declined 75 percent from 2006 to 2007. Some Nigerians are optimistic that the transmission of both wild and vaccine-derived poliovirus can be interrupted in their country and that polio will eventually be eradicated. If this goal is not achieved in 2009, they believe that through continued routine immunization and focused National Immunization Day rounds in areas where immunization levels have historically been very low and resistance to the Polio Eradication Initiative has been high, especially in Kano, Sokoto, Jigawa, and Bauchi States, the last cases of wild poliovirus will be seen in the next few years. One Ahmadu Bello University professor optimistically stated in 2007, "They will eradicate polio in Nigeria, but not for another two to three years, not this year, not next year, but maybe in 2009 or 2010" (interview, Shika, 9 August 2007).[2] If he is correct that wild poliovirus transmission will be terminated, the next step will be to decide what direction to take during the post-transmission era, until the disease's eradication is certified. Several scenarios have been proposed.

Four Post-transmission Scenarios

Four scenarios have been considered for the post-transmission period, after evidence confirms that the transmission of wild poliovirus has been disrupted (Sutter, Cáceres, and Lago 2004). These scenarios include: 1) attenuated oral polio vaccine (OPV) may continue to be used in low-income countries, while inactivated polio vaccine is used in high-income countries; 2) OPV may be universally replaced with inactivated polio vaccine; 3) OPV may be discontinued and optionally replaced with inactivated polio vaccine; or 4) OPV may be discontinued with no plans to replace it with another form of vaccine. Each scenario has its advantages and drawbacks, although some scenarios are more likely than others.

In the first scenario, low-income countries continue to use oral polio vaccine, in order to maintain high levels of immunization that will prevent the spread of subclinical cases of polio, outbreaks of vaccine-derived poliovirus will be possible, so that continued surveillance and lab testing of stool samples from children with acute flaccid paralysis will be required. High-income countries, and eventually middle-income countries, using inactivated polio vaccine would not require this vigilance, although they would incur the cost of inactivated polio vaccine, which is more than five times that of oral polio vaccine. The costs of vaccine, surveillance, and testing would be borne by national governments.

In the second scenario, oral polio vaccine would no longer be used (except in supplemental immunization campaigns) in high-risk, low-income countries, which would switch to the inactivated polio vaccine, already used by middle- and high-income countries. The problem with this approach is not only that the inactivated polio vaccine is expensive, but also that global supplies of it are limited (Miller, Barrett, and Henderson 2006, 1171). It must also be injected by trained medical staff. New developments in its production, however, may address some of these constraints, as economies of scale may allow inactivated polio vaccine manufacturers to reduce prices. Furthermore, inactivated polio vaccines that can be administered intradermally (rather than intramuscularly) may be developed, which will reduce the need for trained personnel; it is also possible that a reduced dose of the inactivated polio vaccine could be combined with vaccines for other early childhood diseases (Ehrenfeld et al. 2008, 1386). Nonetheless, low-income countries would be hard put to fund the purchase of sufficient doses of this vaccine and to train sufficient health workers to administer it.

In the third scenario, low-income countries would stop using oral polio vaccine and rely on surveillance and response, preferably using monovalent oral polio vaccine to address any outbreaks. These countries would also be encouraged to use inactivated polio vaccine. Both middle- and high-income countries would continue routine vaccination with inactivated polio vaccine; all costs would be covered by individual governments. But while surveillance and response may be effective in stopping polio cases exhibiting paralysis, the frequency of subclinical cases of polio, whether due to wild or vaccine-derived virus, make it difficult to know when polio transmission has actually stopped, particularly in growing populations.

Finally, the fourth scenario, in which the oral polio vaccine is discontinued without any replacement, is not a real option, as it would lead to an upsurge in cases of paralytic polio, both in countries where polio had been endemic and elsewhere (Ehrenfeld et al. 2008, 1385–86; Kimman and Boot 2006, 675). Thus only the first three options will be considered in more detail here.

While the first option is the most economical, it risks continued cases of paralytic polio caused by circulating vaccine-derived poliovirus. The second scenario has been discussed by Kimman and Boot (2006), who call for continued high levels of vaccination coverage—ideally 100 percent, using the inactivated vaccine in combination with vaccines for other early childhood diseases, including diphtheria-pertussis-tetanus, measles, rubella, hepatitis B, and *Haemophilus influenzae B*. While they admit that substantial financial costs would be associated with a shift to the use of inactivated polio vaccine as part of a broad program of routine immunization, they argue,

> Because insufficient population immunity could result in the spread of wild-type poliovirus and the emergence of cVDPVs, we do not consider ending the use of OPV to be an option, without first replacing it with IPV. If IPV vaccination is indeed too expensive, impractical, and beyond the reach of many developing countries in the coming years, then, as a second choice option only, it would be prudent to continue the use of OPV, raise its coverage to 100%, and then, if circumstances allow, to slowly replace OPV with IPV. This option would mean that we do not get rid of OPV

quickly, or even that we have to continue its use for ever. However, pursuit of this scenario might be realistic if it helps to improve routine vaccination against a wide range of childhood diseases. (Kimman and Boot 2006, 678)

This argument combines an eradication approach with a long-term control strategy of routine immunization. Others, such as Thompson and Tebbens (2007, 1363), argue that "the intensity of immunization must be increased to achieve eradication [i.e., the termination of transmission], and that even small decreases in intensity could lead to large outbreaks." They believe that low-cost control programs using routine immunization risk continued outbreaks of wild poliovirus and would be more costly in the long run (Roberts 2007a).

Officials at the World Health Organization favor the third option, the discontinuation of oral polio vaccine combined with the optional use of inactivated polio vaccine, because of the risk of vaccine-derived polioviruses (Aylward and Heymann 2005, 776). While WHO will not provide inactivated polio vaccine to individual countries, it will help them assess the costs and benefits of using it. It will also also help them develop and maintain the necessary surveillance and response capability, including building stockpiles of vaccine against need (Aylward and Heymann 2005, 777).

The question of which program is best to pursue in a post-transmission era is difficult to decide. Should polio immunizations be continued for twenty years after the last case of paralytic polio has been identified? If so, should oral vaccine or inactivated vaccine be used—or would it be better to combine inactivated polio vaccine with vaccines against other diseases, to be administered together in a single injection? Should programs for routine immunization against childhood diseases be strengthened? It must be remembered that it is difficult to know whether subclinical cases of polio are still occurring, and that continued use of oral vaccines may lead to the emergence of circulating vaccine-derived polioviruses. All these questions are being discussed and debated (Dobriansky et al. 2007; Rey and Girard 2008; Reynolds 2007).

Yet some are skeptical about whether the transmission of poliovirus can be stopped at all. Arita, Nakane, and Fenner (2006, 852–53) have argued that polio eradication is an unrealistic goal for several reasons, including the large proportion of subclinical cases, the likelihood that the use of oral polio vaccine will lead to outbreaks of vaccine-derived poliovirus, changes in population size and national politics, and the extended period of time during which the Polio Eradication Initiative has been carried out. They have suggested instead a program of "effective control," which would first continue special immunization programs in countries where polio is endemic or is likely to spread. After the global case count falls below five hundred, they recommend the incorporation of polio immunization within a global health strategy which would "integrate immunization, other health interventions, and surveillance in the health systems context."

Some Nigerians are also skeptical about the possibility of ending the transmission of poliovirus in their country and ultimately attaining the goal of polio eradication. For example, one journalist who has written on health issues, including polio, was asked about the prospects for eradication in Nigeria:

> Yes, that [polio eradication] is the projection. [But] it cannot be completely eradicated because if you go to the hinterlands . . . Let me give you an instance. We were in Kebbi with the zonal director in charge of Bauchi. We were at the place where the *malams* gather children; the children were in Islamiyya school. They [the *malamai*] said no. . . . In spite of the NPI officials' pleas that the *malams* allow the children to be immunized, they said, "No." (Interview, Abuja, 17 July 2007)[3]

This man thought that while polio immunization was widely accepted in Nigeria, there were, nonetheless, pockets of resistance, especially in rural areas, which would be very difficult to reach. "Squashing out polio will not be possible, but it will be reduced to a minimum." Others, in Zaria, agree with this assessment:

> It will be difficult to eradicate polio because one needs to reach the grass-roots, which they've still not done. And the small number of confirmed cases of polio, they won't be picking up these "grass-roots" villager cases because they don't go to hospital or clinics and these remote villages, even with oversight [surveillance], they may miss them—or not test them to confirm [it's polio]. The government wants to show that Nigeria is not preventing eradication, so they will underestimate the numbers. (Personal communication, Zaria, August 2007)

> They are doing Polio Plus but it is not clear how they are recording who has received vaccines and how many children have not been vaccinated. . . . I don't think that they will be able to eliminate polio any time soon. (Personal communication, Zaria, August 2006)

> There are still many who do not accept the polio vaccine, it's probably not more than 50–60 percent who have had their children vaccinated for polio. And they are not reporting or finding remaining cases as they don't want the figures to increase. (Personal communication, Zaria, July 2007)

While it may remain difficult to maintain surveillance and accurate record-keeping in the face of pressures to provide the "right" numbers, some Nigerians, like the Ahmadu Bello University professor quoted earlier, are more optimistic, although they may not see primary health care as the answer: "Promoting primary health care will not eradicate polio. . . . But if the momentum [of the campaign] is maintained, maybe [ending polio transmission] by 2011 is more [realistic]" (interview, Shika, 26 July 2006). Others support the improvement of primary health care, arguing for patience and persistence, along with community dialogue, in order to identify the last case of wild poliovirus in Nigeria:

> The main thing is going on slowly, individually, not with mass programs. It didn't work with family planning and there is the same response to

polio. . . . They [health officials] also need to change the way they [parents] think about children. If they are sending their children out as *almajiri* [young male students who beg for their keep], do you think that they will get their children immunized against polio? But I think they will be successful in ridding the country of polio. (Interview, Shika, 24 July 2006)

This long-term approach is viewed optimistically by one young woman from Zaria City who was a polio immunization team member there and who compared people's acceptance of immunization with their eventual acceptance of Western education (*boko*):

Before, when people were asked to come to school [*boko*] to be educated, they used to run away. Before, if they were asked to send their children to *boko*, they would hide their children. But now everyone wants to send their children to school for education. It's the same thing with polio. (Interview, Zaria City, 31 August 2005)

However, one of the principal reasons that Western education has become acceptable is the view that it is something that government provides that is beneficial for children and their futures. In the case of immunization, there are other, more pressing services that parents expect the government to provide for them and their children. Two of these services are the provision of clean drinking water and electricity.

On Water

In the fifteen years since I first moved into two rooms in a family home in Anguwar Kwarbai, the neighborhood surrounding the emir's palace in Zaria City, I've seen many changes in the supply of water and electricity. In 1994, piped water regularly flowed from the compound's tap—at least 3 or 4 times a week. By 2000, it flowed only sporadically. Everyone in the house would stop everything we were doing—day or night—to line up with our buckets at the slightest hint of water gurgling through the pipes. Fortunately, the household was also able to get water from a deep well that the owner had dug years before. Nonetheless, during the summer rainy season, we all set out buckets and basins to catch rainwater as it poured off the metal roof. This was my main source of water during my annual summer residence in the house.

At the end of the dry season in May 2009, the well had dried up. Other sources of water were even more elusive. When I asked about the large metal water tank near the Ban Zazzau Clinic in Zaria City, which had been built during the colonial period, I was told that it no longer functioned. Furthermore, although the World Bank had sponsored a water project in the 1990s that provided boreholes and pumps in another section of Zaria, water from it never reached Zaria City.

When I was visiting Zaria City in February 2008, piped water flowed into the house once—briefly. At that time, I was told by one physician at the Ban Zazzau

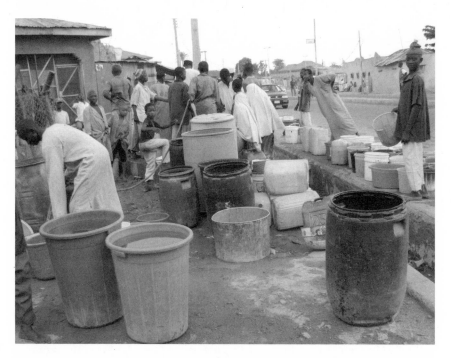

Figure ep.1. Men and boys getting water from a solar-powered water pump in Anguwar Rimi Tsiwa, Zaria City. Photograph by E. P. Renne, Zaria City, 2 June 2009.

Clinic that water had become a major concern of people in Zaria City, as evidenced by the steady flow of children into our compound asking to get water from our well. On one occasion, I noticed a small boy drinking water greedily from a bowl as if he had not drunk any in days. Eventually, the family living in the outer rooms of the compound began locking the entry door in order to stop these incursions. Outside, down the road that intersects the main road through Zaria City, there were at least fifty large plastic jerry cans lined up waiting for their owners, who would arrive in the evening to fill them from a well that dispensed water at sunset each day (fig ep.1). The Kaduna State government had commissioned the building of several wells with solar-powered pumps in Zaria City in 2007, of which this was one, but not all of the wells had been built (Sa'idu 2008).[4] Adults and children organize their days around the time when water flows from these wells or go in search of water from other sources, including ponds and the Kubanni River, the main river in Zaria. As one resident explained,

> Everyone knows that life without water is not feasible. It is better for the government to act now and find a solution to this problem than to come for rescue mission when the looming epidemic blows up. May Allah stop this from happening. People are now taking water without minding the source. Even the streams which people resorted to

as their source of water are now beginning to dry up, exposing the residents to more danger. (Sa'idu 2008, 13)

Such sources of water, which collect runoff from fields and open sewers, are a source of cholera. They may also be a reservoir for poliovirus. The Islamic Development Bank and the Kaduna State Government have recently discussed the provision of a N30 billion (approximately US$235 million) interest-free loan, part of which will be used to rehabilitate the water system in Zaria (Aodu 2008). Despite efforts like this one, water shortages have continued through the summers of 2008 (Balal 2008) and 2009.[5]

*   *   *

Living under these difficult circumstances in Zaria, people may find immunization campaigns such as the Polio Eradication Initiative, planned and carried out by international agencies, immaterial in comparison to everyday concerns such as getting water (Das 1999; Magashi 2005). Dissatisfied by their government's inability to provide water, electricity, and sanitation, along with primary health care, they are apathetic about or distrustful of such campaigns. They may be experiencing "polio fatigue," having become tired of being asked to give their children multiple doses of oral polio vaccine, and they may resist immunization campaigns.

In the U.S., it took time to reduce the incidence of measles, from an average of 450,000 cases annually between 1963 and 1967 (Colgrove 2006, 166), to only sixty-four cases from 1 January to 25 April 2008 (Grady 2008).[6] Several strategies fostered this decline, including the provision of free or subsidized vaccines, better clinic hours, and mandatory school vaccinations. What is not often mentioned is U.S. government support for rural electrification, clean water standards, and local sanitation services. Government commitment to improvements in these basic services as well as primary health care, including a strengthening of routine immunization and education programs, may, over time, result in similar high levels of immunization, as well as a successful conclusion of the Polio Eradication Initiative in Nigeria.[7]

Notes

1. Introduction

1.   It is very uncommon for a fifteen-year-old Nigerian child to get paralytic polio, since by that age most children have acquired natural immunity through environmental exposure and have had an asymptomatic case of polio. However, in Namibia, where wild poliovirus had not been transmitted since 1996, nineteen confirmed cases of wild poliovirus occurred in 2006 in individuals between the ages of fourteen and fifty-one. Fourteen of these cases occurred in individuals between the ages of fifteen and twenty-nine, who presumably had been neither vaccinated nor exposed to the virus as children (CDC 2006a).

2.   In a recent U.S. trial, vaccine manufacturers were accused of causing autism in American children (Harris 2007a).

3.   Farmer (1999, 205) notes a similar dynamic in 1946 in New York City, when a Harlem physician questioned health authorities' focus on polio while many African Americans there were dying from tuberculosis.

4.   Some interviews were conducted in Hausa and were tape-recorded. After recordings were transcribed, a Hausa researcher and I would work on the translations. I have tried to follow the Hausa as closely as possible. I also conducted interviews with some people in English, and have not edited their comments.

5.   For example, the Expert Review Committee on Polio Eradication noted in December 2006 "that the decline in 'noncompliance' had been accompanied by an increase in 'absent children' indicating the need for further investigation" (National Programme on Immunization 2006b, 7). The committee repeated its conclusion almost a year later, in November 2007 (NPHCDA 2007, 2).

6.   This sort of sabotage was also carried out by some health workers, who disliked or had little interest in the program but saw it as a source of income. For example, it was reported that some health workers dumped vaccine when they were unable to meet the day's quota.

7.   A sense of the difficulties faced by polio immunization teams attempting to reach children living in widely dispersed villages and hamlets may be obtained in a WHO video of an Immunization Plus Day in Igabi Local Government Area, Kaduna State, Nigeria, in June 2007 (WHO 2007c).

8.   This decline in the number of confirmed wild poliovirus cases has been accompanied by a significant increase in overall levels of immunization in Nigeria. The interim coordinator of the National Programme on Immunization, Dr. Edugie Abebe, reported that immunization coverage had risen from 35 percent to 75 percent in 2006 (Olayinka 2007b), although WHO and UNICEF report an estimated overall national coverage of 54 percent for the same year (WHO and UNICEF 2007).

9.   According to a survey conducted in Nigeria by UNICEF in 2006, only 54 percent of parents knew that multiple doses of polio vaccine were needed (National Programme on Immunization 2006b, 7).

10. In the Western press, protests against the polio campaign were described almost exclusively as Muslim resistance to an international health intervention (e.g., Altman 2004; McNeil 2005a, 2005b). However, a National Public Radio report, aired on 13 April 2005 (Wilson 2005) and a PBS program (aired on 13 April 2009; Lazaro 2009) presented a more complex picture, from the perspective of Kano health professionals.

11. The Hausa and Fulani are two of the major ethnic groups in Northern Nigeria.

12. The Salafiyya group, a recent offshoot of the Izala movement, established around 2000, supports a return to the religious practices of the time of the Prophet Muhammed.

13. There are also a small numbers of Hausa-Fulani Christians as well as followers of traditional Hausa religion (M. Last 2005).

14. There have been exceptions, of course. Some Christian groups opposed Western medicines during the 1967–70 smallpox campaign in Nigeria (Thompson and Foege 1968).

15. While the colonial government had an Office of Social Welfare within the Ministry of Health to address the problems of the disabled, assistance (with the exception of special education schools) was provided mainly for the blind (Schram 1971).

16. Young girls who are lame have a different social trajectory. They do not commonly beg but rather marry and remain in their husbands' houses, under their care.

17. The higher pay for doing polio vaccinations during National Immunization Days also contributed to health workers' greater interest in the Polio Eradication Initiative than in routine primary health care (Yahya 2007).

18. In 2006, a style of women's dress called Paralyze because of its slanting hemline, which suggested the bodily asymmetry of those with one lame leg, became popular.

2. Smallpox and Polio Histories

1. In 1825, at the behest of the British explorer Hugh Clapperton, Thomas Dickson prepared a list of eighteen different types of medicine—mainly herbal medicines, powders, and metal-based ointments—along with instructions for their use, which were to be given as a gift to the Sheikh of Bornou (Lockhart and Lovejoy 2005, 520–21).

2. *Babba juji* is referred to as the "hairy thorn apple" (*Datura metel*) in Sokoto and Katsina (Dalziel 1916, 11).

3. It is also possible that amulets containing portions of the Qur'an were used for protection against smallpox, as has been documented in Senegal (Marty 1914).

4. This practice was reported as late as the 1960s in more remote villages and hamlets (Fenner et al. 1988, 1163; Herbert 1975).

5. Variolation has been practiced in many parts of the world, including in China by the sixteenth century (Jannetta 2007, 11), Turkey (Jannetta 2007, 15), and the United States (e.g., in Boston, during the 1721 smallpox epidemics there; Fenn 2001, 33). Foy (1915, 256) described the technique of inoculation among the Djen people (in what is now Taraba State) in some detail:

> An incision from half to three-quarters of an inch in length is made through the skin with a razor, a pustule in the patient is opened, and with the end of a straw

some of the lymph is applied to the incision made with the razor. The operator then places a grain of maize into the mouth of the person inoculated and with the end of a fresh straw dipped in the honey he places a drop of honey on the tongue of the individual and subsequently a drop of honey is applied to the seat of the inoculation. The reason for this accessory part of the process of inoculation is as follows: The grain of maize is placed in the mouth of the inoculated person in the belief that when he develops small-pox the vesicles will be large and discrete; the drop of honey is placed on the tongue so that the eruption may come out quickly and contents of the vesicles will be clear like honey in the comb.

6. By 1908, "there were sixty-three medical officers in Nigeria in government service" (Schram 1971, 141), although these doctors were primarily concerned with maintaining the health of the expatriate population.

7. According to Schram (1971, 159), "in 1907 an Ordinance was passed forbidding the worship of the smallpox juju (god, or orisha), and heavy fines were inflicted on many of its priests." As late as 1957, priests of Shopona continued this practice in Ibadan, in southwestern Nigeria.

8. While this number of individuals may have been vaccinated, figures are not given for the number of vaccinations which "took." One officer noted that it was difficult to get people to return to have their scars checked because they feared being revaccinated.

9. Smallpox inoculation was documented during the colonial period (Herbert 1975, 544) among groups in southern Kaduna State, such as the Katab, and in Taraba State, such as the Jukun. Meek (1931, 312) describes Jukun inoculation, in which a piece of straw was used to transfer lymph from a pustule from someone who had had smallpox for eight or nine days to a slit made in the left forearm of the patient. Herbert mentions that Hausa migrants in Ghana performed inoculation there, although it had been made illegal by British colonial officials; in Northern Ghana (at Yendi), "two mallams were carrying out arm-to-arm inoculation during an outbreak of smallpox there" (Herbert 1975, 546).

10. In 1961, Adeniyi-Jones (1961, 321) reported that deaths from smallpox "are now relatively rare in Lagos owing to the wide acceptance of vaccination." While in 1958 there were 579 cases reported at Lagos General Hospital, with 12 percent case mortality, by 1960 there were only thirty-two cases, with six deaths.

11. This ordinance also prohibits "arm to arm vaccination," presumably referring to local methods of inoculation.

12. He is referring to the 1949–51 cerebrospinal meningitis epidemic in Northern Nigeria (Horn 1951).

13. This may have been the case in an example in Ningi, a village southeast of Kano, in August 1971, described by Besmer (1977, 3–4):

> The ritual subject, a Warji woman from Katanga town, was said to have led an untroubled life, even though she had recently been estranged from her husband and had experimented with prostitution. Living with her own family, she awoke one morning with a numbness in the left side of her body. It soon became worse, and she found herself a cripple, her left hand and foot useless. Her family was justifiably alarmed and sought to have her cured as an outpatient at the dispensary. The dispenser either failed to cure her or refused to take her case, so the family sought help elsewhere. Their inquiries led them to Ningi town and, eventually, to its *Sarkin Bori* who claimed to understand her illness.

During her seclusion the neophyte was treated with various medicines derived mostly from plant sources which she either drank, washed with, was rubbed with, or inhaled smoke. She was taught to demonstrate possession-trance for not only the Black Tall-Woman who had caused her illness but for fourteen other spirits either related to this principal spirit or important in her special circumstances.

The woman was nearly completely cured of her paralysis by the end of the eighth day, after which she became an adept of Mai Baku, the bowman spirit, which had been associated with her father's family (Besmer 1977, 4).

14. In a piece on *bori* worship published in the *Official Gazette* in 1910, one colonial official noted that "His Excellency the Governor [Lord Lugard] directs that Residents are to urge on the Native Administrations the desirability of suppressing whenever possible all practices connected with 'Bori'" (Alexander 1910). An example from Gwari in southern Kaduna Province, southwest of Zaria, suggests the subversive nature of this spirit cult. During the colonial period, the pantheon of *bori* spirits began to include British administrative officials and medical workers. A woman was possessed by the *bori* spirit known as Bature Gwari (the white man from Gwari), which appeared before the village head, who had forbidden bori worship in the town. Because the spirit appeared as a white man, it was outside of the village head's jurisdiction (Smith 1954, 287n17).

15. The West African population was considered to have "natural immunity" (Gelfand and Miller 1956), hence the director of medical services, Northern Region, reported that

> the Nigerian born and living in Nigeria has a very high rate of immunity against poliomyelitis and their vaccination is unnecessary, except in certain circumstances. The expatriate community, however, is only partially immune and those adults who are not immune are exposed to a serious risk of contracting serious poliomyelitis. (D. J. M. Mackenzie, 19 July 1956, in Outbreak of Smallpox, Nigerian National Archives)

16. The chief medical adviser advocated immunization prior to coming to Nigeria: "In the circumstances, and until more is known of the epidemiology of poliomyelitis in Nigeria, you may wish to inform your directorate of our advice that your officers and their families should be vaccinated in their countries of origin rather than in Nigeria" (N. Leitch, 19 September 1956, in Salk Anti-poliomyelitis Vaccine, Nigerian National Archives).

17. Livingston (2005, 157, 271n74) describes a similar dynamic in Lesotho and South Africa, where "most of the polio patients doctors identified were European."

18. An additional serological study was carried out in 1959 in Oloibiri, a Niger Delta village or town, where high levels of type 1 polio antibodies were found (Anonymous 1961).

19. It is not clear from this article how the diagnosis was confirmed.

20. In Northern Nigeria, this inspection depended on having women as well as men health workers.

21. Health workers found evidence of variolation on the left arms of some adult villagers, although there was no evidence of recent inoculation (Pifer and Adeoye 1968).

22. Alhaji Nuhu Bamalli, the Magajin Garin Zazzau, served as a cabinet minister in the Ministry of Foreign Affairs (in 1960), as a member of the Constitution

Assembly (in 1967), and as the chairman of the Jama'atu Nasril Islam, Kaduna State (in 1988).

3. Politics and Polio in Nigeria

1. From January to March 2009, there were 1,728 cases of cerebrospinal meningitis in Kaduna State, as reported by the Kaduna State Commission for Health (*Daily Trust* 2009a). In Nigeria as a whole, there were 40,000 cases and 1,900 deaths, "the biggest [outbreak] in five years," according to the European Union regional information officer (*Daily Trust* 2009b).

2. The lack of sustained support for a national primary health care system—it was left to the budgetary discretion of local governments—is due to political and economic factors, including payments on an accumulated foreign debt of US$30 billion (Polgreen 2005; see also World Bank 2008).

3. According to a report by Feilden Battersby Analysts (2005, 2), both the National Programme on Immunization and the National Primary Health Care Development Agency were parastatals "under the control of the Permanent Secretary in the Federal Ministry of Health and hence the Minister of Health." However, since the directorships of both were presidential appointments, they had considerable independence from these officials.

4. There were 2,971 confirmed new polio cases worldwide in 2000 (WHO 2007a).

5. In 1995, even before the implementation of the Polio Eradication Initiative and eight years before the Kano vaccination boycott, one Ahmadu Bello University physician observed, "A lot of people [in Zaria] don't get the Expanded Programme on Immunisation vaccine now because they believe that family planning drugs, fertility control drugs, are incorporated in it" (Renne 1996, 133).

6. One UNICEF official suggested that there was a vindictive motive behind this move, because "a wealthy Kano doctor who was both head of a campaign to impose Islamic law in northern Nigeria and a candidate for a top job in the national health department" was passed over for the appointment (Dugger and McNeil 2006, A14). Some local people, nonetheless, realized that some individuals who spoke out against polio immunization had their own political agendas. One man who had followed the advice of a local Muslim leader (and university lecturer) bitterly remarked, "He misled us," after his child was paralyzed with polio (interview, Samaru, 12 July 2005).

7. A story in the *Daily Trust* also reported that no hormones were found in the vaccine. Skepticism about this finding is evident from the remark "that no pressure has been brought to bear on [the investigators] with regard to this issue" (Alimi 2003). In fact, traces of estradiol were found in the vaccine. One Muslim woman leader observed that asserting that no hormones had been found was a mistaken strategy; instead, officials should have tried to explain why such traces were not harmful (personal communication). According to the health columnist for the *Daily Trust*, Aminu Magashi, "the bone of contention in Nigeria is an issue, not of rumor or suspicion, but of whether the Estradiol level can cause harm or not, and the majority of the polio stakeholders are of the belief that it will cause no harm" (Magashi 2004).

8. As has been noted, the availability of viable vaccine has been a continual problem (FBA Health Systems Analysts 2005). In his study of a village in Tarauni

LG, Kano State Local Government, Muhammed (2003) cited "no vaccine" as one of the primary reasons that villagers' children were not being immunized. One Kano journalist noted that a friend "took his infant daughter for DPT [diptheria-pertussis-tetanus] immunization more than 10 times, . . . no allocation" (Magashi 2003), although there appears to be some variability in clinic services.

Between January and May 2006, 95 percent of local government areas reported that they had no Bacillus Calmette-Guérin (tuberculosis) vaccine in stock; 84 percent had no oral polio vaccine; 76 percent had no hepatitis B vaccine; and 68 percent had no DPT vaccine (National Programme on Immunization 2006a, 6). This lack of vaccine may partially explain the high number of confirmed wild poliovirus cases in 2006.

9.   Indeed, some believe that vaccines and injections may cause paralysis.

10.   In 2009, some primary and nursery school principals allowed parents to submit letters requesting that their children not be immunized during National Immunization Day exercises (personal communication, Zaria, 2009).

11.   Yahya (2007, 195) noted that it was not only women with only Islamic education, but also those with Islamic and Western education, who distrusted vaccination team members entering their houses, exemplified by one woman's response: "When asked whether she would allow her son to be vaccinated by the door-to-door vaccinators, as opposed to having her son vaccinated in a private clinic, she said she would not take that risk with her son."

12.   One reason for this woman's hostile response was that previously, when she had taken her daughter for measles vaccination, the child had become very sick with measles. However, she subsequently allowed her children to be vaccinated in order to obtain a bednet (personal communication, Zaria, 2006).

13.   There was some suspicion that women wanted bednets in order to sell them. One WHO official said that health workers had begun to remove the plastic packaging of nets to prevent this practice (personal communication, Kaduna, August 2007). However, in a small survey conducted in Zaria City in 2007, women who had received nets through the polio campaign were either using them themselves or had given them to relatives. Sales of bednets through local markets, when they occur, do so at a higher level, through local government health officials (personal communication, Zaria, July 2007).

14.   For example, the monies allocated to local governments for National Immunization Days were not only being mismanaged at the local level, but were also "being siphoned off, all along the way" (personal communication, Samaru, 2006; see also Mbakwem and Smith 2009).

15.   The COMPASS program was developed in 2004 by USAID to actively involve community members in health initiatives (COMPASS 2007a); it ended in 2009 (Rabiu 2009).

4. Islam and Immunization in Northern Nigeria

All quotations from the Qur'an are taken from Ahmed Ali's translation (Al-Qur'an 1994).

1.   See Martin 1994 for a discussion of American views of the workings of the immune system.

2. Last (1967, 5) has noted that the belief in *aljanu* existed before the jihad and continued afterward, reinforced by mentions of them in the Hadith and in the writings of Sheikh Usman dan Fodio himself.

3. This man and several others argued that the decrease in disease in the West was caused by such factors as good nutrition and improved hygiene, rather than by specific medical interventions such as antibiotics and vaccines. This argument was made popular by René Dubos (1959).

4. He is referring to sura 95, verse 4.

5. In a June 2007 trial in Washington, D.C., a group of parents of autistic children sought damages from the U.S. government for allowing vaccines to contain thimerosal, a preservative that contains ethyl mercury, although this preservative is no longer used (Harris 2007a). The parents lost their case and major studies have found no link between vaccine use and autism, yet some parents continue to question the safety of vaccines and refuse to obtain immunizations for their children (Harris 2007b).

6. The Hausa word *allura* means both hypodermic needles and those used for sewing. It also has magical uses: *allura harbin* are supernatural needles sent to harm someone (Newman and Newman 1979, 4; see also M. Last 2004, 723).

7. Several anthropological studies have examined interpretations of injections: see Bierlich 2000; Reeler 2000; Samuelsen 2001; van Staa and Hardon 1996; and Whyte and van der Geest 1994.

8. The cardiologist who treated her diagnosed her as having suffered a minor stroke which had temporarily reduced blood circulation in the brain, causing temporary paralysis which could be ameliorated through physical therapy.

9. The site of one of the early colonial clinics in Zaria City is called *babban dodo*, big masquerade or spirit. I was told that the name reflects local views of colonial medical officials as frightening, powerful beings. It is also possible that the name refers to the British missionary Dr. Walter Miller, who lived in the area in the 1930s (personal communication; Miller n.d.).

10. Alhaji Abubakar Gumi, the founder of the reformist Islamic movement known as Izala, made regular radio and later television addresses (*tafsir*) discussing the Qur'an and the Hadith, which Izala leaders see as constituting the basis of proper Muslim conduct.

11. In their 2005 study of routine immunization services in Nigeria, the consulting firm Feilden Battersby Analysts (FBA Health Systems Analysts 2005, 30) examined a 2003 survey carried out by the National Programme on Immunization which found that in 30 out of 37 states, "vaccine not available" was the reason parents cited most for not immunizing their children, followed by "place of immunization too far" (23 out of 37 states) and being "unaware of the need for immunization" (20 out of 37 states).

12. However, these figures actually compared favorably with the *Nigeria Demographic and Health Survey 2003,* which found that 40.5 percent of 356 children in northwestern Nigeria had no immunization prior to its survey (National Population Commission and ORC Macro 2004, 130; see also Bonu, Rani, and Razum 2004).

13. It is possible that these figures reflect poor reporting practices; also some children may have been vaccinated through the Ahmadu Bello University Teaching Hospital and these figures may not have been merged.

14. The Zaria Local Government health coordinator noted, "Blood samples from three affected children in Wuciciri ward were taken to Kaduna two weeks ago for

proper diagnosis" (*Daily Trust* 2007). See Marks and Andersson 1988 for another example of government downplaying death rates.

15. Etkin, Ross, and Muazzamu (1990, 921) describe the treatment of measles using traditional medicine and also how the concepts of bitterness and coolness frame ideas about appropriate pharmaceutical treatments.

16. Distrust of the MMR vaccine (for mumps, measles, and rubella) was also mentioned in the June 2007 vaccine trial in Washington, D.C. Lawyers for the family of one child argued that the MMR vaccine caused a "chronic measles infection that damaged her central nervous system" and that the thimerosal in it "damaged her immune system, making it impossible for her to fight the infection" (Harris 2007a). The controversy in the UK over the MMR vaccine and its possible connection to autism had been reported in Nigeria in a March 2004 issue of the *Daily Trust* (2004b).

17. Colgrove (2006, 15) describes a similar situation in the U.S. in the 1950s, where vaccination coverage was lowest in poor areas. Subsequently, U.S. health officials focused on "improving the health care delivery system to make it more equitable and accessible." Colgrove provides a detailed discussion of the uses of coercion (requiring immunization before children could attend public school) and persuasion (e.g., publicity campaigns) to increase immunization levels in the U.S.

18. After an outbreak of vaccine-derived poliovirus in Kano, a Muslim cleric who had formerly rejected the Polio Eradication Initiative but had come to accept it noted that "the state government was mostly responsible for the problems it faced. 'We should thank our foreign friends for coming to help,' he said. 'But we should ask, where is our government in all this? If this came about because of unsanitary conditions, isn't that the government's responsibility?'" (Walker 2007a).

19. He is referring to the United States National Security Council's National Security Study Memorandum 200 (see USAID 1994).

20. Four of the countries (or areas of the countries) in the world where wild poliovirus remains endemic are predominantly Muslim, and health officials have called for the Gulf States to help fund the continuing effort to eradicate polio worldwide (McNeil 2005b). Yet it is important to note that many Islamic nations which have ended the transmission of wild poliovirus have strong primary health care and immunization programs.

5. Polio, Disability, and Begging

1. This way of viewing disability became apparent in a discussion about polio in Zaria City in which a visiting U.S. graduate student asked if being lame was stigmatizing. When she explained that people in the U.S. would try to hide such an impairment, one of the two Zaria women who were present expressed her shock that someone would try to reject "what God had given."

2. The practice of begging and staying with Zongo chiefs has been abandoned in Accra, where it is now expected that the disabled will be trained to work or will be supported by the government (interview, Accra, 25 May 2009; personal communication, 2009). See Weiss 2007 for a detailed discussion of Islamic leaders' views on begging, government efforts to eliminate begging, and the relationship between begging and poverty in Ghana.

3. One such group was described by Abner Cohen in his 1962–63 study of the large Hausa migrant community in Ibadan in southern Nigeria. Cohen mentions the Ibadan "Chief of the Lame, *Sarkin Guragu*," "who holds a special title and who is officially turbaned by the Chief of the Quarter in a special public ceremony" (1969, 45, 44).

4. Ogala (1971, 6) mentions interviewing nine polio-disabled beggars as part of his study, but did not find any groups of polio-disabled beggars. This observation corresponds with Kungiyar Guragu members' statement that their organization in Zaria was founded fourteen years after Ogala conducted his research there. Most of the disabled people who were organized in groups in Zaria at that time either had leprosy (49 percent of his sample) or were blind (31 percent).

5. This raises the question of whether the disabled prefer partners with similar conditions or whether lame women are less eligible marriage partners (Fassin 1991). Some deaf parents in the U.S. use genetic testing to ensure that they will have deaf children (Sanghavi 2006).

6. Similarly, in her study of Yoruba parents' views on handicapped children, Okunade (1981, 192) found that the educated elite were more willing to have a child marry into a family with a handicapped member than were those with little education.

7. As the Sarkin Kutare in Sabon Gari put it, "We are not poor financially, we feed our families and some of us are even able to do more. Our main problem is that we are looked upon as a strange group of people by the public and therefore we have no place in the society" (Ogala 1971, 6–7).

8. A second settlement, Alheri Special Village, was founded in Yangoje in the Kwali area council of Abuja as part of this rehabilitation plan. The village is intended for beggars with leprosy; it has modern housing, water, electricity, and a hospital but only a primary school and few opportunities for employment (J. Abubakar 2007, 37).

9. See also Bankole 2007, which discusses Rotary programs for the physically disabled in southern Nigeria.

10. In Jigawa State (to the east of Kano), the newly elected governor, Alhaji Sule Lamido, has also recently authorized a census of the disabled with the goal of rehabilitating beggars through training and the provision of stipends in order to eliminate begging there, which will be made illegal (A.-R. Abubakar 2008).

11. The Hausa is

> *Matukar da musakai barkatai, da makaho ko da makauniya.*
> *Ba mahallai nasu a Hausa duk, Ba mai tanyonsu da dukiya.*
> *Birni kauye da garuwa duk suna yawo a Nijeriya.*
> *Kai Bahaushe bashi da zuciya, za ya sha kunya nan duniya!* (Furniss 1996, 226).

6. Polio in Northern Nigeria and Northeastern Ghana

1. This figure does not include the sixty-two vaccine-derived polio cases in Nigeria in 2008.

2. See Wilks 1965 for a discussion of the origins of Islam in Northeastern Ghana and its relationship with Hausa religious leaders and Northern Nigeria.

3. The Northern Region of Ghana is also similar to Northern Nigeria, with its high mortality rates for children under five and low levels of contraceptive use by

married women (Ghana Statistical Service, Ghana Health Service, and Macro International 2009; National Population Commission and ORC Macro 2004).

4. The last indigenous Ghanaian case of wild poliovirus was confirmed in 2000 in Bole District, Northern Region. All three confirmed cases in the Northern Region in 2003—one each in Yendi, East Mamprussi, and East Gonja Districts—were attributed to Northern Nigeria. All of the cases in 2008 were traced to Northern Nigeria as well.

5. Funding was provided by the World Bank, DANIDA (the Danish International Development Association), DFID (the British Department for International Development), the European Union, USAID, and the Dutch government, and WHO, UNICEF, and the CDC provided logistical assistance.

6. Initially the trivalent oral polio vaccine was used. However, since the seven confirmed cases of polio were caused by type 1 poliovirus, in November health officials switched to the monovalent type 1 polio vaccine, which is more effective than the trivalent one (Grassley et al. 2007).

7. The Northern Region also has the most cases of guinea worm, the object of another international eradication effort in Ghana. Of 147 cases reported nationally between January and March 2009, all but one were found in the Northern Region (Nurudeen 2009), reflecting the lack of piped water there. The preponderance of cases also reflects relative unconcern with guinea worm, which, as Bierlich (1995, 507) notes, "is not considered a health problem demanding particular attention or explanation." It is possible that polio is viewed in a similar way.

8. A violent conflict known as the "Guinea Fowl War" broke out in Yendi District in February 1994 between the Konkomba and Dagomba. It continued through May 1994, when the federal government established a negotiation team to address the underlying causes of the violence (Mahama 2003, 104).

9. Health workers in East and West Mamprussi also experienced violence themselves. In West Mamprussi, one health worker was attacked by robbers and his motorcycle stolen, and another was killed on the East Mamprussi border (interview, Tamale, 22 May 2009).

10. The taxi fare between Kano, Nigeria, and Maradi, Niger, was N1,200 in 2009, slightly less than the N1,500 fare from Kano to Abuja, the Nigerian federal capital.

11. It is sometimes difficult even to determine what country a polio case is in. In early 2009, the WHO polio website reported one case in Ghana which was subsequently attributed to Togo (interview, Tamale, 22 May 2009).

12. The problems posed by the mobility of people and of infectious disease was also noted during the Smallpox Eradication Program, first when an outbreak of cases in southern Kaduna State was linked to railroad workers and later when migratory Fulani families fell through the cracks of local health jurisdiction (Smallpox eradication and measles control campaign, Nigerian National Archives; Pifer and Adeoye 1968).

13. The death rate of children under five in Ghana dropped from 155 deaths per thousand in 1983–87 to 88 in 2003–2007. However, there are considerable differences in under-five mortality rates between regions in the more recent period, with the Greater Accra Region having an under-five mortality rate of 68, while the Northern Region's rate is 123, the highest in the country (Ghana Statistical Service, Ghana Health Service, and Macro International 2009, 117).

14. The 2003 Nigerian Demographic Survey reported an infant mortality rate ranging from 129 to 136 per thousand in Northern Nigeria, which actually represented an increase over the rates reported in the 1990 survey (National Population Commission and ORC Macro 2004, 109).

7. The Ethics of Eradication

1. The ethics of cultural relativism itself have been criticized by anthropologists when local practices involve significant physical harm. Although such criticisms are not the focus of this analysis, see Das 1999 for a discussion of the ethics of cultural relativism in anthropological research.

2. See Meskell and Pels 2005 for examples of different ethical approaches within anthropology. Some anthropologists who are also medical doctors have particular ethical conundrums (Harper 2007). As a cultural anthropologist, I am ethically responsible for protecting study participants from harm—social, physical, or psychological—and for respecting those with whom I interact. This responsibility also entails masking people's identities and places that might give these identities away without their permission, as well as providing study communities with copies of all subsequent publications. As a member of the University of Michigan academic community, I am also responsible for obtaining approval for all research projects involving human subjects from the university's Institutional Review Board.

3. Sura 2, verse 233 enjoins parents to care for their children to the best of their ability:

> Mothers should breast feed their children two full years, provided they want to complete the nursing. The family head must support women and clothe them properly. Yet no person is charged with more than he can cope with. No mother should be made to suffer because of her child, nor family head because of his child.

4. When questioned by Jane Lenzer, a writer for the *British Medical Journal*, about this dosage, "Pfizer acknowledged to the *BMJ* that it used a low dose of ceftriaxone—33 mg/kg. When asked why a low dose was chosen, Pfizer's spokesperson, Bryant Haskins, said that full dose shots were too 'painful' for the children and made it hard for them to walk." Lenzer then contacted the U.S. Food and Drug Administration about whether this low dosage had been approved and was told that drug trial protocol was not public information. However, "the FDA spokesperson acknowledged that the recommended daily dose of ceftriaxone for the treatment of meningitis is 100 mg/kg" (Lenzer 2007, 1181).

5. The official transcript of the hearing was published in full in the Northern Nigerian newspaper *The Daily Trust* in late May and early June 2006.

6. By comparing the molecular composition of vaccine-derived poliovirus case isolates with that of the Sabin attenuated poliovirus used in oral polio vaccine, specialists are able to determine approximately when and where the original oral polio vaccine dose, from which the infectious virus derived, was given (Kew et al. 2004).

7. One case of circulating vaccine-derived poliovirus was reported on the WHO website in 2006 and cases were reported in the *Polio Lab Network* (WHO 2007c) in April 2007, although this report would not likely have been seen by

nonspecialists (McNeil 2007). There were also two journal articles describing cases of type 2 vaccine-derived poliovirus, one in 2001, published in 2003 (Adu et al. 2003) and one case in 2002, published in 2007 (Adu et al. 2007), although the 2001 case was seen at the time as an isolated incident.

8. This lack of knowledge among health workers about the outbreak is not surprising, considering the general misperceptions of the oral polio vaccine held by some of them. Interviews of 265 health workers who participated in the third round of the 2003 Sub-National Immunization Days in Gombe Local Government Area revealed that "22 (8.3%) perceived that OPV was harmful due to repeated administration, 26 (9.8%) perceived that OPV had sterility property, contained harmful materials 14 (5.3%) and HIV 11 (4.2%)" (Arulogun and Obute 2007).

9. For those who followed the biweekly reports of acute flaccid paralysis and confirmed wild poliovirus case counts posted on the WHO website, it was puzzling to see one case of circulating vaccine-derived poliovirus mentioned on 14 September 2006 and then to learn in 2007 that there were actually sixty-nine such cases between January 2006 and 17 August 2007, according to data provided by the CDC (CDC 2007b). While annual data on circulating vaccine-derived poliovirus cases in Nigeria was revised on the WHO website in 2008, the discretionary use of numbers lends credence to those who have questioned the accuracy of WHO data (e.g., FBA Health Systems Analysts 2005, 22). Indeed, data collection and misrepresentation have been an ongoing problem, as one University of Ibadan professor observed:

> The most difficult thing is a lack of data . . . and we don't have a system for birth and deaths or disease outbreak monitoring. That is the problem. I can give you an example. In 1975, I used to keep a register when I was in the system. I recorded 350 new cases of polio at University College Hospital in Ibadan and reported all of them, on signed forms to the Public Health Office at the Secretariat. When the summary came out [of events] that occurred in 1975, they said there were only twenty-five cases of polio! So it's been a long-time problem. (Interview, Ibadan, 22 February 2008)

10. For others, such as Arita (cited in Arita, Nakane, and Fenner 2006, 852), ten to fifteen years is an acceptable period. Yekutiel's shorter time frame reflects his argument that some diseases can be effectively regionally eradicated.

11. The term "elimination" is sometimes used interchangeably with "eradication," and although this term too has been variously interpreted, according to Miller, Barrett, and Henderson (2006, 1165) it refers to the "cessation of transmission of an organism throughout a country or region," and such cessation requires continued interventions, such as immunization, to prevent the reemergence of the disease.

12. Ironically, it was Governor Shekarau who halted the distribution of polio vaccine in Kano State in 2003. Although he has backed the campaign since July of the following year, Kano State had a third of the cases of wild poliovirus in Nigeria in 2008 (*Nation* 2008).

13. For example, the Expert Review Committee noted with some consternation in March 2008 that "of the 4 remaining polio endemic countries in the world, Nigeria now accounts for nearly 90% of the type 1 cases, reporting 40 cases by 11 March 2008" (National Primary Health Care Development Agency 2008).

14. Some question whether this perspective is appropriate in the first instance (Farmer 1999).

15. In 2008, three cases of circulating vaccine-derived poliovirus (derived from oral polio vaccine) were identified in Ethiopia and fourteen cases were found in the Democratic Republic of Congo (CDC 2009a).

16. The last cases of indigenous wild poliovirus were identified in The Gambia in 2000 (WHO 2009; see also chapter 6, note 4).

17. The Hausa is *To, idan magana cewa na arzikin kasa ya dore ne. To, ka gaya ma yawa a duniya ka kasa zana zanne, na wajen basu kawo ba, kuma na cikin gurgu ne. Ka tara kudi junguru amma bamu daina talauci ba.*

18. For example, one report stated that "at one point in early 2005 a pin board could not be screwed to the wall until the CE/NC [Awosika] had approved the proposed location of the pin board." Authority for the financial management of the Initiative was centralized and opaque, masking inaccuracies, e.g., "errors of additions . . . amounting to billions of Naira" in the program budget (FBA Health Systems Analysts 2005, 24, 26). Awosika resigned on 12 December 2005. In 2008, newspaper stories outlined the privatization of several government companies (Gulloma 2008) and the sale of properties to political allies (A.-R. Abubakar 2008).

Epilogue

1. In response to this concern and as part of the international measles initiative, nationwide measles immunization days were held in 2005 and 2008.

2. He meant that the transmission of wild poliovirus would be stopped. The conflation of eradication with the termination of wild poliovirus transmission is not uncommon, as was discussed in chapter 7.

3. A similar example was cited in Bauchi State in 2008. According to Ruby Rabiu (2008a), Dr. Lawal Hadejia, director of the National Primary Health Care Development Agency, Bauchi State, "said the resistance was so pronounced in such areas because, according to him, some religious and opinion leaders were against administering vaccines. According to him, various meetings were held with these highly respected men to educate and sensitise them about the importance of the immunization to eradicate polio, but all to no avail." This resistance may have diminished somewhat in the wake of the initiative of the Sultan of Sokoto, Alhaji Muhammad Sa'ad Abubakar, who organized a committee of fourteen Northern Nigerian traditional rulers to address it on 15 June 2009 (Mudashir 2009).

4. According to one resident in Tudun Jukun, workers began to dig a hole there in late 2007 but it was never completed. One of the state assemblymen from the area, who was organizing the project, said that the contractor was responsible for the delay (Sa'idu 2008, 13).

5. I was told that on Sunday, 24 May 2009, young men, their bodies covered with sand, marched through the streets of Zaria City chanting, "*Ba ruwa, ba wuta!*" (No water, no light). When they arrived at the Emir's palace, the Emir counseled them to have patience (see also H. Muhammad 2009). The next day, another protest by young men at Sabon Gari-Zaria took place, with four deaths reported (I. Musa et al. 2009).

6.   Health officials are concerned about recent measles outbreaks in the U.S. In 2000, there were no cases reported; the sixty-four reported in the first four months of 2008 are more than were reported in all of 2007 (Grady 2008).

7.   Singh et al. (2007) make a similar argument for India, where wild poliovirus is also endemic and where environmental health problems hamper polio eradication efforts.

Bibliography

Aaby, Peter. 1995. Assumptions and contradictions in measles and measles immunization research: Is measles good for something? *Social Science & Medicine* 41 (5): 673–86.

———. 2004. Being wrong in the right direction? *Lancet* 364 (9438): 984.

Abdalla, Ismail. 1991. Neither friend nor foe: The *malam* practitioner—'*Yan bori* relationship in Hausaland. In *Women's Medicine: The Zar-Bori Cult in Africa and Beyond,* ed. I. M. Lewis, A. Al-Safi, and S. Hurreiz, 37–48. Edinburgh: Edinburgh University Press for the International African Institute.

———. 1997. *Islam, Medicine, and Practitioners in Northern Nigeria.* Lewiston, N.Y.: Edwin Mellen Press

Abdullah, Nuruddeen. 2009a. Kano Trovan drug—Pfizer to pay N11.2bn compensation—How Gowon, Carter negotiated settlement. *Daily Trust,* 1 March, http://www.dailytrust.com, accessed 1 March 2009.

———. 2009b. Pfizer compensation and the challenge facing the authorities. *Daily Trust,* 5 April, http://www.dailytrust.com, accessed 5 April 2009.

Abdullahi v. Pfizer, Inc. 2005. 01 Civ. 8118 (WHP), United States District Court for the Southern District of New York, 2005 U.S. Dist. LEXIS 16126, 9 August 2005.

Abdulmalik, Yahaya. 2008. Grange: No sacred cow, AC insists. *Daily Trust,* 28 March, http://www.dailytrust.com, accessed 28 March 2008.

Abubakar, Abdul-Rahman. 2008. Sale of VP's houses: Rules were flouted, el-Rufai admits. *Daily Trust,* 30 April, http://www.dailytrust.com, accessed 6 May 2008.

Abubakar, Ahmed. 2007. Lamido to abolish begging in Jigawa. *Daily Trust,* 28 May.

Abubakar, Jibrin. 2007. We are dying—FCT beggars. *Daily Trust,* 21 August, http://www.dailytrust.com, accessed 10 Nov. 2007.

Achebe, Chidio. 2004. The polio epidemic in Nigeria: A public health emergency. 14 July. http://www.nigeriavillagesquare.com/articles/Chidi-C<->Achebe/the-polio-epidemic-in-nigeria.html, accessed 12 December 2009.

Adeniyi-Jones, O. 1961. The control of communicable diseases in pre-school children in Lagos. *West African Medical Journal* 10 (4): 320–26.

Adu, Festus, Jane Iber, David Bukbuk, Nicksy Gumede, Su-Ju Yang, Jaume Jorba, Ray Campagnioli, et al. 2007. Isolation of recombinant type 2 vaccine-derived poliovirus (VDPV) from a Nigerian child. *Virus Research* 127:17–25.

Adu, Festus, Jane Iber, Tekena Harry, Cara Burns, Oluseyi Oyedele, Johnson Adeniji, Mubarak Ossei-Kwasi, et al. 2003. Some genetic characteristics of sabin-like poliovirus isolated from acute flaccid paralysis cases in Nigeria. *African Journal of Biotechnology* 2 (11): 460–64.

Alabi, O. 1995. Expansion on immunization. *Daily Sketch,* 22 June.

Alexander, D. 1910. Notes on Bori. *Official Gazette (Northern Nigeria)* 11, supplement no. 8: xxi. Nigerian National Archives, Kaduna.

Alimi, Zainab. 2003. No reproductive hormones in polio vaccine—National Hospital. *Daily Trust,* 18 November.

Aliyu, Ruqayyah. 2008. Kano records low interest in immunization. *Daily Trust,* 25 June, http://www.dailytrust.com, accessed 25 June 2009.

Al-Jawziyya, Ibn Qayyim. 2001. *The Prophetic Medicine.* Karachi: Hafiz and Sons.

Al-Qur'an. 1994. Translated by Ahmed Ali. Princeton, N.J.: Princeton University Press.

Altman, Lawrence K. 2004. Polio cases in West Africa may thwart W.H.O. plan. *New York Times,* 11 January.

Alubo, S. Ogoh. 1990. State violence and health in Nigeria. *Social Science & Medicine* 31 (10): 1075–84.

Amwe, Ayuba O. 2007. Screening of children living with disabilities for admission to Kaduna State Special Education School (KASSES) and Integration Centres for 2007/2008 session, CNC/1.427/VOL III. Unpublished document, Ministry of Education, Kaduna State.

Anamzoya, Alhassan S. 2004. A sociological enquiry into the 2002 Dagbon chieftaincy conflict in the northern region of Ghana. M. Phil. thesis, Department of Sociology, University of Ghana-Legon.

Anand, Sudhir, Fabienne Peter, and Amatya Sen, eds. 2004. *Public Health, Ethics, and Equity.* Oxford: Oxford University Press.

Andrews, Jason. 2006. Research in the ranks: Vulnerable subjects, coercible collaboration, and the hepatitis E vaccine trial in Nepal. *Perspectives in Biology and Medicine* 49 (1): 35–51.

An-Nawawi. 1991. *Forty Hadith.* Kaduna.

Anonymous. 1955. *Report on the Enquiry Into Begging and Destitution in the Gold Coast, 1954.* Kumasi[?]: Department of Social Welfare and Community Development.

Anonymous. 1961. Discussion, session no. 3. *West African Journal of Medicine* 10 (4): 229.

Anonymous. 1990. Editorial: Structural adjustment and health in Africa. *Lancet* 335 (8694): 885–86.

Anonymous. 1996. What has Nigeria lost? *Newswatch* 24 (4): 8–11.

Anonymous. 2007. Progress towards poliomyelitis eradication in Nigeria, January 2005 to December 2006. *Weekly Epidemiological Record* 82 (13): 105–16.

Aodu, AbdulRaheem. 2007a. 1000 disabled, *almajirai* receive free computer training. *Daily Trust,* 19 July.

———. 2007b. JNI backs WHO to meet polio eradication target. *Daily Trust,* 20 July.

———. 2007c. Measles outbreak kills over 50 in Zaria. *Daily Trust,* 5 December.

———. 2008. IDB to rehabilitate Zaria waterworks. *Weekly Trust,* 6 Aprilhttp://www.dailytrust.com, accessed 6 April 2008.

Arita, Isao, Miyuki Nakane, and Frank Fenner. 2006. Is polio eradication realistic? *Science* 312 (5775): 852–54.

Arulogun, Oyedunni S., and J. A. Obute. 2007. Health workers' perception about the supplemental immunization activities in Gombe Local Government Area, Gombe State. Abstract. http://www.ncbi.nlm.nih.gov/pubmed/17874492, accessed 12 December 2009. *African Journal of Medicine and Medical Sciences* 36 (1): 65–70.

Attah, James O. 2003. Assessment of polio eradication strategies in Zaria Local Government Area of Kaduna State. MPH/DCM, Department of Community Medicine. Zaria: Ahmadu Bello University.

Ayensu, Edward. 1978. *Medical Plants of West Africa.* Algonac, Mich.: Reference Publications.

Aylward, R. Bruce, and David Heymann. 2005. Can we capitalize on the virtues of vaccines? Insights from the Polio Eradication Initiative. *American Journal of Public Health* 95 (5): 773–78.

Aylward, R. Bruce, Roland Sutter, and David Heymann. 2005. OPV cessation—the final step to a "polio-free" world. *Science* 310:625–26.

Babadoko, Sani. 2003. Sharia body wants polio vaccination suspended. *Daily Trust,* 28 July.

———. 2007a. Closure of textiles threat to security in Kaduna—Yakowa. *Daily Trust,* 4 Nov. http://www.dailytrust.com, accessed 11 December 2007.

———. 2007b. Measles death toll rises to 200 in Zaria. *Daily Trust,* 10 December. http://www.dailytrust.com, accessed 13 December 2007.

Babadoko, Sani, and Musa U. Kazaure. 2004. Polio vaccine contaminated—JNI reports. *Daily Trust,* 26 January.

Bako, C. A. 1978. Status of immunization in children under 5 in Ahmadu Bello University Teaching Hospital, Zaria. Long essay, Department of Community Medicine, Ahmadu Bello University, Zaria.

Balal, Atka. 2008. Zaria: Empty wells, silent taps. *Daily Trust,* 4 July. http://www.dailytrust.com, accessed 4 July 2008.

Bamalli, Nuhu. 1961. *Bala da Babiya: Lafiya Uwar Jiki.* Zaria: Gaskiya Corporation.

Bankole, Ade. 2007. Rotary: Treat the disabled fairly. *Nation,* 21 June.

Barrett, Ronald. 2006. Dark winter and the spring of 1972: Deflecting the social lessons of smallpox. *Medical Anthropology* 25 (2): 171–91.

Barrett, Scott. 2004. Eradication versus control: The economics of global infectious disease policies. *Bulletin of the World Health Organization* 82 (9): 683–88.

Barth, Heinrich. 1857. *Travels and Discoveries in North and Central Africa.* Vols. 1–3. New York: Harper and Brothers.

Beauchamp, Dan, and Bonnie Steinbock, eds. 1999. *New Ethics for the Public's Health.* New York: Oxford University Press.

Bego, Abdullahi. 2007 We certified polio vaccine safe since 1964—Professor Umaru Shehu. *Daily Trust,* 14 March.

Benjamin, Sunday. 2005. NPI boss sacked. *Daily Trust,* 14 November.

Besmer, Fremont. 1977. Initiation into the Bori cult: A case study in Ningi Town. *Africa* 47 (1): 1–13.

Bierlich, Bernhard. 1995. Notions and treatments of guinea worm in Northern Ghana. *Social Science & Medicine* 41 (4): 501–509.

———. 2000. Injections and the fear of death: An essay on the limits of biomedicine among the Dagomba of Northern Ghana. *Social Science & Medicine* 50 (5): 703–13.

———. 2007. *The Problem of Money: African Agency and Western Medicine in Northern Ghana.* New York: Berghahn Books.

Blume, Stuart. 2006. Anti-vaccination movements and their interpretations. *Social Science & Medicine* 62 (3): 628–42.

Bonu, Sekhor, Manju Rani, and Timothy Baker. 2003. The impact of the national polio immunization campaign on levels and equity in immunization coverage: Evidence from rural North India. *Social Science & Medicine* 57 (10): 1807–19.

Bonu, Sekhor, Manju Rani, and Oliver Razum. 2004. Global public health mandates in a diverse world: The polio eradication initiative and the expanded programme on immunization in sub-Saharan Africa and South Asia. *Health Policy* 70 (3): 327–45.

Bradley, Peter. 2000a. Application of ethical theory to rationing in health care in the UK: A move to more explicit principles? In *Ethics in Public and Community Health,* ed. Peter Bradley and Amanda Burls, 3–19. London: Routledge.

———. 2000b. Should childhood immunization be compulsory? In *Ethics in Public and Community Health,* ed. Peter Bradley and Amanda Burls, 167–76. London: Routledge.

Bradley, Peter, and Amanda Burls. 2000. *Ethics in Public and Community Health.* London: Routledge.

Brenzel, Logan, Lara J. Wolfson, Julia Fox-Rushby, Mark Miller, and Neal A. Halsey. 2006. Vaccine-preventable diseases. In *Disease Control Priorities in Developing Countries,* 2nd ed., ed. Dean T. Jamison, Joel Breman, Anthony Measham, George Allenyne, Mariam Claeson, David Evans, Prabhat Jha, Annne Mills, and Philip Musgrove, 389–411. New York: Oxford University Press.

Butcher, James. 2008. Polio eradication nears the end game. *Lancet Neurology* 7 (4): 292–93.

Castro, Arachu, and Merrill Singer, eds. 2004. *Unhealthy Health Policy: A Critical Anthropological Examination.* Walnut Creek, Calif.: Altamira Press.

CDC (Centers for Disease Control and Prevention). 2005. Progress toward poliomyelitis eradication—Nigeria, January 2004–July 2005. *Morbidity and Mortality Weekly Report,* 54 (35): 873–77.

———. 2006a. Outbreak of polio in adults—Namibia, 2006. *Morbidity and Mortality Weekly Report* 55 (44): 1198–1201.

———. 2006b. Resurgence of wild poliovirus type 1 transmission and consequences of importation—21 countries, 2002–2005. *Morbidity and Mortality Weekly Report* 55 (6): 145–50.

———. 2007a. Laboratory surveillance for wild and vaccine-derived polioviruses—Worldwide, January 2006–June 2007. *Morbidity and Mortality Weekly Report,* 56 (37): 965–69.

———. 2007b. Update on vaccine-derived polioviruses—Worldwide, January 2006–August 2007. *Morbidity and Mortality Weekly Report,* 56 (38): 996–1001.

———. 2009a. Circulating vaccine-derived poliovirus. Website of the Global Polio Eradication Initiative. http://www.polioeradication.org/content/general/cvdpv_count .pdf, accessed 8 July 2009.

———. 2009b. Website of the Global Polio Eradication Initiative (17 June), http://www .polioeradication.org, accessed 18 June 2009.

———. 2009c. Progress toward interruption of wild poliovirus transmission—Worldwide, 2008. *Morbidity and Mortality Weekly Report,* 58 (12): 308–12.

Cheng, Maria. 2007. Officials say drug caused Nigeria polio. AP, Yahoo.com News, 5 October. http://www.yahoo.com, accessed 5 October 2007.

Clapperton, Hugh. 1829. *Journal of the Second Expedition into the Interior of Africa.* London: Cass. 1966.

Cockburn, A. 1963. *The Evolution and Eradication of Infectious Diseases.* Baltimore: Johns Hopkins University Press. Quoted in Yekutiel 1980, 6.

Cohen, Abner. 1969. *Custom and Politics in Urban Africa.* Berkeley: University of California Press.

Colgrove, James. 2006. *State of Immunity: The Politics of Vaccination in Twentieth-Century America.* Berkeley: University of California Press; New York: Milbank Memorial Fund.

Collis, W. R., O. Ransome-Kuti, M. E. Taylor, and L. E. Baker. 1961. Poliomyelitis in Nigeria. *West African Medical Journal* 10:217–22.

Community Participation for Action in the Social Sector (COMPASS). 2007a. About COMPASS. http://www.compassnigeria.org/, accessed 10 November 2007.

———. 2007b. Success story: Polio victims adopt enterprising ways to sustain change initiatives. July. http://www.compassnigeria.org/site/PageServer?pagename= Success_Stories_200707_Polio_Enterprising_Initiatives, accessed 10 November 2007.

Compulsory Vaccination in Northern Provinces. 1945. KAD-MOH, file 420, Nigerian National Archives, Kaduna.

Cooper, Barbara. 1997. *Marriage in Maradi.* Portsmouth, N.H.: Heinemann.

da Costa, Gilbert. 2007. New measles outbreak reported in Nigeria. *Voice of America,* 5 December. http://www.voanews.com/english/2007-12-05-voa38.cfm, accessed 11 December 2007.

Daily Trust. 2004a. Kano imports polio vaccine from Indonesia. 17 May.

———. 2004b. Oral polio vaccine is safe—Sultan of Sokoto. 22 March.

———. 2007. Measles kills 150 in Zaria. 8 December. http://www.dailytrust.com, accessed 13 December 2007.

———. 2009a. Meningitis kills 80 in Kaduna in three months. 23 April. http://www.dailytrust.com, accessed 23 April 2009.

———. 2009b. Nigeria records biggest meningitis epidemic. 23 April. http://www.dailytrust.com, accessed 23 April 2009.

Daiyabu, Mohammed. 1977–78. Immunisation in the Tudum Wada Under-5s Clinic, 1976, Zaria. Long essay, Department of Community Medicine, Ahmadu Bello University, Zaria.

Dalziel, John. 1916. *A Hausa Botanical Vocabulary.* London: T. Fisher Unwin.

Daniel, S. Ola. 1978. An epidemiology of physical conditions of destitute (beggars) in Lagos. *Journal of Tropical Medicine and Hygiene* 81:80–83.

Das, Veena. 1999. Public good, ethics, and everyday life: Beyond the boundaries of bioethics. *Daedalus* 128 (4): 99–133.

Delaney, Carol. 1987. Symbols of procreation. In: *Turkic Culture: Continuity and Change,* ed. Sabri M. Akural, 41–48. Bloomington: Turkish Studies, Indiana University.

Denham, Dixon, and Hugh Clapperton. 1826. *Narrative of Travels and Discoveries in Northern and Central Africa in the Years 1822, 1823, and 1824.* London: J. Murray.

Dobriansky, Paula, Julie Gerberding, Kent Hill, and J. Stephen Morrison. 2007. Is polio eradication possible? A discussion of the global effort to eradicate polio, recent setbacks, and opportunities for success. Video and transcript of a panel discussion at the Center for Strategic and International Studies, Washington, D.C., 1 May 2007. http://www.kaisernetwork.org/healthcast/csis/01may07, accessed 4 May 2007.

Dowdle, Walter R. 1998. The principles of disease elimination and eradication. In *Global Disease Elimination and Eradication as Public Health Strategies,* ed. Goodman et al., 22–25. *Bulletin of the World Health Organization* 76, supplement 2.

Dubos, René. 1959. *Mirage of Health.* Garden City, N.Y.: Anchor Books.

Dugger, Celia. 2007. Polio fight gets $200 million injection. *New York Times,* 20 November.

Dugger, Celia, and Donald G. McNeil, Jr. 2006. Rumor, fear and fatigue hinder final push to end polio. *New York Times,* 20 March.

Dyer, Owen. 2005. WHO's attempts to eradicate polio are thwarted in Africa and Asia. *British Medical Journal* 330 (14 May): 1106.

Eades, Jeremy. 1980. *The Yoruba Today.* Cambridge: Cambridge University Press.

Edlich, Richard F., Dana M. Olson, Brianna. M. Olson, Jill A. Greene, K. Dean Gubler, Kathryne L. Winters, Angela R. Kelley, L. D. Britt, and William B. Long III. 2007.

Update on the National Vaccine Injury Compensation Program. *Journal of Emergency Medicine* 33 (2): 199–211.

Ehrenfeld, Ellie, Roger I. Glass, Vadim I. Agol, Konstantin Chumakov, Walter Dowdle, T. Jacob John, Samuel L. Katz, Mark Miller, Joel G. Breman, John Modlin, and Peter Wright. 2008. Immunisation against poliomyelitis: Moving forward. *Lancet* 371 (9621): 1385–87.

Ejembi, Clara, Elisha Renne, and Haruna A. Adamu. 1998. The politics of the 1996 cerebrospinal meningitis epidemic in Nigeria. *Africa* 68 (1): 118–34.

Ekanem, E. 1988. A 10-year review of morbidity from childhood preventable diseases in Nigeria: How successful is the expanded programme of immunization (EPI)? *Journal of Tropical Pediatrics* 34:323–28.

Ekpo, M. D. 1975–76. Current state of immunity in Kaduna population. Long essay, Department of Community Medicine, Ahmadu Bello University, Zaria.

Employment of Disabled People. 1952–53. MOH-Kaduna, vol. 1, file 4020, Nigerian National Archives, Kaduna.

Etkin, Nina L. 1981. A Hausa herbal pharmacopoeia: Biomedical evaluation of commonly used plant medicines. *Journal of Ethnopharmacology* 4:75–98.

———. 1992. "Side effects": Cultural constructions and reinterpretations of Western pharmaceuticals. *Medical Anthropology Quarterly* 6 (2): 99–113.

Etkin, Nina, Paul Ross, and Ibrahim Muazzamu. 1990. The indigenization of pharmaceuticals: Therapeutic transition in rural Hausa Land. *Social Science & Medicine* 30:919–28.

Familusi, Julius B., and V. A. O. Adesina. 1977. Poliomyelitis in Nigeria: Epidemiological pattern of the disease among Ibadan children. *Journal of Tropical Paediatrics and Environmental Child Health* 23:120–24.

Farmer, Paul. 1999. *Infections and Inequalities: The Modern Plagues.* Berkeley: University of California Press, 2001.

———. 2005. *Pathologies of Power: Health, Human Rights, and the New War on the Poor.* Berkeley: University of California Press.

Fassin, Didier. 1991. Handicaps physiques, practiques economiques et strategies matrimoniales au Senegal. *Social Science & Medicine* 32 (3): 267–72.

Federal Ministry of Health, Nigeria. 1991. *Expanded Program on Immunization: The National Coverage Survey, Preliminary Report, 18 April 1991.* Lagos: Federal Ministry of Health.

FBA Health Systems Analysts. 2005. The state of routine immunization services in Nigeria and reasons for current problems. Bath: FBA Health Systems Analysts. http://www.technet21.org/backgrounddocs.html, accessed 15 August 2005. (This web page has been discontinued; a revised version of the report is available at http://www.technet21.org/Tools_and_resources/pdf_file/State_of_Immunization_in_Nigeria.pdf, accessed 30 October 2009.)

Feldman-Savelsberg, Pamela, Flavien Ndonko, and Bergis Schmidt-Ehry. 2000. Sterilizing vaccines, or the politics of the womb: Retrospective study of a rumor in Cameroon. *Medical Anthropology Quarterly* 14 (2): 159–79.

Fenn, Elizabeth. 2001. *Pox Americana: The Great Smallpox Epidemic of 1775–1982.* New York: Hill and Wang.

Fenner, Frank, Donald A. Henderson, Isao Arita, Z. Jezek, and I. D. Ladnyi. 1988. *Smallpox and Its Eradication.* Geneva: World Health Organization.

Ferguson, James. 1994. *The Anti-politics Machine.* Minneapolis: University of Minnesota Press.

Fine, Paul E. M., and Ulla Kou Griffiths. 2007. Global poliomyelitis eradication: Status and implications. *Lancet* 369 (9570): 1321–22.

Foege, William H., J. D. Millar, and Donald A. Henderson. 1975. Smallpox eradication in West and Central Africa. *Bulletin of the World Health Organization* 52 (2): 209–22.

Foster, Stanley, and E. Ademola Smith. 1970. The epidemiology of smallpox in Nigeria. *Journal of the Nigerian Medical Association* 7 (3): 41–45.

Foy, Andrew. 1915. Inoculation of small-pox as a prophylactic measure as practiced by the natives at Djen in Nigeria. *Journal of Tropical Medicine and Hygiene* 18:255–57.

Francis, Thomas, Jr., J. Napier, R. Voight, F. Hemphill, H. Wenner, R. Korns, M. Boisen, E. Tolchinsky, and E. Diamond. 1957. *Evaluation of the 1954 Field Trial of Poliomyelitis Vaccine; Final Report.* Ann Arbor, Mich.: Edwards Brothers.

Fredrickson, Doren F., Terry Davis, Connie Arnold, Estela Kennen, Sharon Humiston, J. Thomas Cross, and Joseph Bocchini. 2004. Childhood immunization refusal: provider and parent perceptions. *Family Medicine* 36:431–39.

Fry, David. 1965. Some complications of illicit injections. *West African Medical Journal* 14:167–69.

Furniss, Graham. 1996. *Poetry, Prose and Popular Culture in Hausa.* Washington, D.C.: Smithsonian Institution Press.

Gelfand, Henry, and Max Miller. 1956. Poliomyelitis in Liberia. *American Journal of Tropical Medicine* 5:791–96.

Geurts, Kathryn. 2002. *Culture and the Senses: Bodily Ways of Knowing in an African Community.* Berkeley: University of California Press.

Ghana News Agency. 2008. Polio case detected in Yendi. *Myjoyonline News,* 17 October. http://news.myjoyonline.com/health/200810/21745.asp, accessed 31 December 2008.

———. 2009. Five million children to be immunized against polio. *Ghana Business News,* 11 February. http://ghanabusinessnews.com/2009/02/11/five-million-children-to-be-immunized-against-polio, accessed 8 April 2009.

Ghana Statistical Service, Ghana Health Service, and Macro International. 2009. *Ghana Maternal Health Survey 2007.* Calverton, Md.: Ghana Statistical Service, Ghana Health Service, and Macro International.

Ghana Statistical Service, Noguchi Memorial Institute for Medical Research, and ORC Macro. 2004. *Ghana Demographic and Health Survey 2003.* Calverton, Md.: Ghana Statistical Service, Noguchi Memorial Institute for Medical Research, and ORC Macro.

Goffman, Erving. 1963. *Stigma: Notes on the Management of Spoiled Identity.* New York: Simon and Schuster.

Goodman, R. A., K. L. Foster, F. L. Trowbridge, and J. P. Figueroa, eds. 1998. *Global Disease Elimination and Eradication as Public Health Strategies. Bulletin of the World Health Organization* 76, supplement 2.

Gouffé, Claude. 1966. Manger et boire en Haoussa. *Revue de l'École nationale des langues orientales* 3:77–111.

Grady, Denise. 2008. U.S. sounds an alert as measles flares. *New York Times,* 2 May.

Grassley, Nicholas C., Jay Wenger, Sunita Durrani, Sunil Bahl, Jagadish M. Deshpande, Roland R. Sutter, David L. Heymann, and R. Bruce Aylward. 2007. Protective efficacy of a monovalent oral type 1 poliovirus vaccine: A case-control study. *Lancet* 369 (9570): 1356–62.

Greenough, Paul. 1995. Intimidation, coercion and resistance in the final stages of the South Asian Smallpox Eradication Campaign, 1973–1975. *Social Science & Medicine* 41 (5): 633–45.

Guardian. 1997. Government plans immunization days. 9 Jan.

Gulloma, Abdullahi. 2006. Polio: NPI boss appeals for cooperation. *Daily Trust,* 6 January.

———. 2008. Anti-Obasanjo strike next week. *Daily Trust,* 2 May. http://www.dailytrust.com, accessed 2 May 2008.

Hallah, Tashikalmah. 2005. LG to jail parents who reject polio immunization. *Daily Trust,* 11 August.

———. 2008. No steady power supply until 2012—Rep. *Daily Trust,* 17 June. http://www.dailytrust.com, accessed 28 June 2008.

Hardon, Anita, and Stuart Blume. 2005. Shifts in global immunisation goals (1984–2004): Unfinished agendas and mixed results. *Social Science & Medicine* 60: 345–56.

Harper, Ian. 2007. Translating ethics: Research public health and medical practices in Nepal. *Social Science & Medicine* 65 (11): 2235–47.

Harris, Gardiner. 2005. Five cases of polio in Amish group raise new fears. *New York Times,* 8 November.

———. 2007a. Opening statements in case on autism and vaccinations. *New York Times,* 12 June.

———. 2007b. Vaccine compound is harmless, study says, as autism debate rages. *New York Times,* 27 September.

Haruna, Mohammed. 2005. The NPI: Why Dr. Dere Awosika should go. *Daily Trust,* 30 November.

Hassan, Maryam G. 2007. Abuja beggars back to business. *Daily Trust,* 18 August.

Henderson, Donald A. 1998. The siren song of eradication. *Journal of the Royal College of Physicians of London* 32 (6): 580–84.

———. 1999. Lessons from the eradication campaigns. *Vaccine* 17, supplement 3: S53–S55.

Henry, P. 1955. Report on the use of a sample of dried lymph. MOH-Kaduna, file 52B, vol. 3, 1953–1955, Nigerian National Archives, Kaduna.

Herbert, Eugenia. 1975. Smallpox inoculation in Africa. *Journal of African History* 16 (4): 539–59.

Heymann, David L., and R. Bruce Aylward. 2004. Eradicating polio. *New England Journal of Medicine* 351 (13): 1275–77.

Holland, Stephen. 2007. *Public Health Ethics.* Cambridge: Polity Press.

Holzer, Brigitte, Arthur Vreede, and Gabriele Weigt, eds. 1999. *Disability in Different Cultures: Reflections on Local Concepts.* New Brunswick, N.J.: Transaction Publishers.

Horn, D. W. 1951. The epidemic of cerebrospinal fever in the Northern Provinces of Nigeria, 1949–1950. *Journal of the Royal Sanitation Institute* 71:573–88.

———. 1952. Notes on smallpox in Nigeria. Vaccination Campaign Reports, 1949–1954. KAD-MOH 5/1, file 52, vol. 1, Nigerian National Archives, Kaduna.

Hull, Harry. 2004. Poliomyelitis. In *Principles of Medicine in Africa,* 3rd ed., ed. Eldryd Parry, Richard Godfrey, David Mabey, and Geoffrey Gill, 696–701. Cambridge: Cambridge University Press.

Hull, Harry, and R. Bruce Aylward. 2001. Progress towards global polio eradication. *Vaccine* 19:4378–84.

Ibrahim, Yusha'u A. 2003. C'ttee assures of thorough investigation on polio vaccination. *Daily Trust,* 9 October.

Idris, Hamza. 2006. NPI predicts eradication of polio by 2007. *Daily Trust,* 20 July.

Ingstad, Benedicte, and Susan Reynolds Whyte, eds. 1995. *Disability and Culture.* Berkeley: University of California Press.

IRIN News. 2007a. Niger-Nigeria: Polio down 80 percent with remaining cases blamed on borders. *IRIN NEWS,* 17 August. http://www.irinnews.org/Report.aspx?ReportID=73771, accessed 13 December 2009.

Jakeway, F. D. 1945. An ordinance to amend the vaccination ordinance. *Nigerian Gazette,* 1945, no. 16:273–75.

James, William. 1891. The moral philosopher and the moral life. In *Essays on Faith and Morals,* 184–215. New York: New American Library, 1962.

Jannetta, Ann. 2007. *The Vaccinators: Smallpox, Medical Knowledge, and the "Opening" of Japan.* Stanford, Calif.: Stanford University Press.

Janzen, John. 1978. *The Quest for Therapy in Lower Zaire.* Berkeley: University of California Press.

Jegede, Ayodele Samuel. 2007. What led to the Nigerian boycott of the polio vaccination campaign? *PLoS Medicine* 4 (3): e73, doi:10.1371/journal.pmed.0040073.

Jinju, Muhammadu. 1990. *African Traditional Medicine: A Case Study of Hausa Medicinal Plants and Therapy.* Zaria: Gaskiya Press.

Johnston, Harry A. S. 1966. *A Selection of Hausa Stories.* Oxford: Clarendon Press.

Joseph, Hir. 2009a. Makurdi, environs not fully covered in polio immunization—parents. *Daily Trust,* 10 April. http://www.dailytrust.com, accessed 10 April 2009.

———. 2009b. Parents complain of immunization's poor coverage. *Daily Trust,* 11 June.

Kar, Anita. 2007. Correspondence. *Lancet* 370 (9582): 131–32.

Karofi, Hassan. 2008a. Kano places priority on polio eradication. *Daily Trust,* 7 April. http://www.dailytrust.com, accessed 14 April 2008.

———. 2008b. Pfizer: Kano govt., victims reject $10m offer. *Daily Trust,* 9 July. http://www.dailytrust.com, accessed 9 July 2008.

Kazaure, M. 2004. Kano rejects FG, JNI reports. *Weekly Trust,* 18 March/

Kew, Olen, Peter Wright, Vadim Agol, Francis Delpeyroux, Hiroyuki Shimizu, Neal Nathanson, and Mark Pallansch. 2004. Circulating vaccine-derived polioviruses: Current state of knowledge. *Bulletin of the World Health Organization* 82 (1): 16–23.

Kimman, Tjeerd, and Hein Boot. 2006. The polio eradication effort has been a great success—let's finish it and replace it with something even better. *Lancet Infectious Diseases* 6 (10): 675–78.

Knobler, Stacey, Joshua Lederberg, and Leslie A. Pray, eds. 2002. *Considerations for Viral Disease Eradication: Lessons Learned and Future Strategies.* Washington, D.C.: National Academy Press.

Kuhn, Philip. 1990. *Soulstealers.* Cambridge, Mass.: Harvard University Press.

Kunitz, Stephen. 1987. Explanations and ideologies of mortality patterns. *Population and Development Review* 13 (3): 379–408.

———. 2006. *The Health of Populations: General Theories and Particular Realities.* New York: Oxford University Press.

Kwaru, Mustapha. 2007. Polio association happy with govt. *Sunday Trust,* 9 September. http://www.sunday.dailytrust.com, accessed 7 October 2007.

Last, Alex. 2007. Vaccine-linked polio hits Nigeria. *BBC News,* 10 October. http://news.bbc.co.uk/2/hi/africa/7037462.stm, accessed 10 October 2007.

Last, Murray. 1967. A note on attitudes to the supernatural in the Sokoto jihad. *Journal of the Historical Society of Nigeria* 4:3–13.

————. 1981. The importance of knowing about not knowing. *Social Science & Medicine* 15B (3): 387–92.

————. 2004. Hausa. In *Encyclopedia of Medical Anthropology: Health and Illness in the World's Cultures*, ed. Carol R. Ember and Melvin Ember, 2:718–29. New York: Kluwer Academic.

————. 2005. Religion and healing in Hausaland. In *African Religion and Social Change: Essays in Honor of John Peel*, ed. T. Falola, 549–62. Durham, N.C.: Carolina Academic Press.

————. 2007. Muslims and Christians in Nigeria: An economy of political panic. *Round Table* 96 (392): 605–16.

————. 2008. The search for security in Northern Nigeria. *Africa* 78 (1): 41–63.

Lazaro, Fred de Sam. 2009. Health workers renew fight against polio in Kano. *The Online NewsHour, with Gwen Ifill,* 13 April. http://www.pbs.org/newshour/bb/africa/jan-june09/nigeria_04-13.html, accessed 20 April 2009.

Leach, Melissa, and James Fairhead. 2007. *Vaccine Anxieties: Global Science, Child Health and Society.* London: Earthscan.

Lenzer, Jane. 2007. Nigeria files criminal charges against Pfizer. *British Medical Journal* 334 (7605): 1181.

————. 2009. Appeals court rules that Nigerian families can sue Pfizer in U.S. *British Medical Journal* 338:b458.

Lentz, Carola. 2006. *Ethnicity and the Making of History in Northern Ghana.* Edinburgh: Edinburgh University Press for the International African Institute.

Lewin, Tamara. 2001. Families sue Pfizer on test of antibiotic. *New York Times,* 30 August.

Livingston, Julie. 2005. *Debility and the Moral Imagination in Botswana.* Bloomington: Indiana University Press.

Lockhart, Jamie, and Paul Lovejoy, eds. 2005. *Hugh Clapperton into the Interior of Africa: Records of the Second Expedition, 1825–1827.* Leiden: Brill.

Lubeck, Paul. 1985. Islamic protest under semi-industrial capitalism: 'Yan Tatsine explained. *Africa* 55 (4): 369–89.

Magashi, Aminu. 2003. Dr. Murzi, UNICEF and polio in Nigeria (I). *Daily Trust,* 24 June.

————. 2004. Polio spread: An appeal to W.H.O. and Kano. *Daily Trust,* 29 June.

————. 2005. Haruna, NPI, and under five mortality. *Daily Trust,* 27 December.

Mahama, Ibrahim. 2003. *Ethnic Conflicts in Northern Ghana.* Tamale: Cyber Systems.

Mahmud, Abdulmalik. 1985. Rehabilitation of destitute: The duty of Muslim community (2). *New Nigerian,* 16 August.

Mansoor, F., S. Hamid, T. Mir, R. Abdul Hafiz, and A. Mounts. 2005. Incidence of traumatic injection neuropathy among children in Pakistan. *Eastern Mediterranean Health Journal* 11(4): 798–804.

Marks, Shula, and Niel Andersson. 1988. Typhus and social control. In *Disease, Medicine, and Empire: Perspectives on Western Medicine and the Experience of Western Expansion,* ed. Roy MacLeod and Milton Lewis, 257–83. London: Routledge.

Martin, Emily. 1994. *Flexible Bodies: Tracking Immunity in American Culture, from the Days of Polio to the Age of AIDS.* Boston: Beacon Press.

Marty, Paul. 1914. Les amulets musulmanes au Senegal. *Revue du monde musulman* 37:319–68.

Marx, Arthur, Jonathan Glass, and Roland Sutter. 2000. Differential diagnosis of acute flaccid paralysis and its role in poliomyelitis surveillance. *Epidemiologic Reviews* 22 (2): 298–316.

Mbakwem, Benjamin, and Daniel Smith. 2009. "Returned to sender": Corruption in international health in Nigeria. In *The Practice of International Health,* ed. D. Perlman and A. Roy, 217–30. Oxford: Oxford University Press.

McNeil, Donald, Jr. 2005a. African strain of polio virus hits Indonesia. *New York Times,* 3 May.

———. 2005b. Health officials say Gulf nations should give more to fight polio. *New York Times,* 7 May.

———. 2007. Polio in Nigeria traced to mutating vaccine. *New York Times,* 11 October.

———. 2008a. Eradicate malaria? Doubters fuel debate. *New York Times,* 4 March.

———. 2008b. Polio spreads to new countries and increases where it's endemic. *New York Times,* 28 October.

Meek, Charles K. 1931. *Tribal Studies in Northern Nigeria.* London: K. Paul, Trench, Trubner and Co.

Meskell, Lynn, and Peter Pels. 2005. *Embedding Ethics: Shifting Boundaries of the Anthropological Profession.* Oxford: Berg.

Miles, William F. C. 1994. *Hausaland Divided: Colonialism and Independence in Nigeria and Niger.* Ithaca, N.Y.: Cornell University Press.

Miller, Mark, Scott Barrett, and Donald A. Henderson. 2006. Control and eradication. In *Disease Control Priorities in Developing Countries,* 2nd ed., ed. Dean Jamison, Joel Breman, Anthony Measham, George Allenyne, Mariam Claeson, David Evans, Prabhat Jha, Annne Mills, and Philip Musgrove, 1163–76. New York: Oxford University Press.

Miller, Walter. N.d. *Walter Miller, 1872–1952: An Autobiography.* Zaria: Gaskiya Corporation.

Mudashir, Ismail. 2009. Sultan constitutes committee on polio. *Daily Trust,* 16 June.

Muhammad, Garba D. 2003. The debate goes on. *Weekly Trust,* 13–19 December.

Muhammad, Hamisu. 2009. Zaria riots not for power blackout—PHCN. *Daily Trust,* 28 May. http://www.dailytrust.com, accessed 28 May 2009.

Muhammed, Mukhtar Bala. 2003. Factors responsible for rejection of polio immunization campaign: A case study of Tarauni LGA, Kano State. Master's thesis in public health, Ahmadu Bello University.

Muhammad, Rakiya. 2009. Kebbi records 15 fresh polio cases. *Weekly Trust,* 13 June.

Musa, Ibraheem, Yusuf Aliy, Isa Sa'idu, and Hamisu Muhammad. 2009. Protest against power blackout: 4 die in Zaria riots. *Daily Trust,* 26 May. http://www.dailytrust.com, accessed 4 August 2009.

Musa, Jamilah. 2004. Four million Kano children for immunization. *Daily Trust,* 26 July.

Musa, Njadvara. 2008. Immunization: Report resisting parents. *Daily Trust,* 4 March.

The Nation. 2008. Nigeria to immunize 4.6 million children against polio. 6 July. http://thenationonlineng.com/, accessed 8 July 2008.

National Planning Commission and UNICEF. 2001. *Children's and Women's Rights in Nigeria: A Wake-Up Call; Situation Assessment and Analysis, 2001.* Abuja: National Planning Commission and UNICEF-Nigeria.

National Population Commission and ORC Macro. 2004. *Nigeria Demographic and Health Survey 2003.* Calverton, Md.: National Population Commission and ORC Macro.

National Primary Health Care Development Agency. 2007. 13th meeting of the Expert Review Committee (ERC) on polio eradication in Nigeria. Abuja, 8–9 November. http://www.polioeradication.org/content/meetings/13thERCMeetingFinalReportNov2007.pdf, accessed 26 November 2007.

———. 2008. 14th meeting of the Expert Review Committee (ERC) on polio eradication and routing immunization in Nigeria. Jos, 12–13 March. http://www.polioeradication.org/content/meetings/14thERCMeetingFinalReportMar2008.pdf, accessed 30 August 2008.

National Programme on Immunization, Nigeria. 2006a. 10th meeting of the Expert Review Committee (ERC) on polio eradication in Nigeria. Kano, 12–13 July. http://www.polioeradication.org/content/meetings/10thERCMeetingFinalReport Jul2006.pdf, accessed 15 May 2007.

———. 2006b. 11th meeting of the Expert Review Committee (ERC) on polio eradication in Nigeria. Abuja, 7–8 December. http://www.polioeradication.org/content/meetings/11thERCMeetingFinalReportDec2006.pdf, accessed 25 October 2007.

Nations, Marilyn, and Christina Monte. 1996. "I'm not dog, no!" Cries of resistance against cholera control campaigns. *Social Science & Medicine* 43 (6): 1007–24.

Needham, Gill. 2000. Using a citizens' jury to involve the public in a decision about priorities: A case study. In *Ethics in Public and Community Health,* ed. Peter Bradley and Amanda Burls, 45–58. London: Routledge.

Needham, Rodney. 1971. *Rethinking Kinship and Marriage.* London: Tavistock.

Newman, Paul, and Roxana Newman. 1979. *Modern Hausa-English Dictionary.* Ibadan: University Press.

New Nigerian. 1969. Vaccination exercise begins. Sept. 12.

New York Times. 2006. Panel to back 3rd term for leader. 10 March.

NPHCDA. *See* National Primary Health Care Development Agency.

Nichter, Mark. 1995. Vaccinations in the Third World: A consideration of community demand. *Social Science & Medicine* 41 (5): 617–32.

———. 1996. Vaccinations in the Third World: A consideration of community demand. In *Anthropology and International Health: African Case Studies,* ed. M. Nichter and M. Nichter, 329–65. Amsterdam: Gordon and Breach.

Ninji, Haruna A. 2006. "Ba mu yarda tazarce ba." Audiocassette recording, purchased in Zaria, August 2007.

Nsaful, J. E. 1967. District Intelligence Report, Yendi. File NR68/3/27, Ghanaian National Archives, Tamale.

Nurudeen, Salifu. 2009. Guinea worm eradication makes progress. *Daily Graphic,* 15 May.

Nwuga, Vincent, and Tokunbo Odunowo. 1978. Some clinical characteristics of children with paralytic poliomyelitis referred for physiotherapy. *Journal of Tropical Medicine and Hygiene* 81:84–87.

Obadare, Ebenezer. 2005. A crisis of trust: History, politics, religion and the polio controversy in Northern Nigeria. *Patterns of Prejudice* 39 (3): 265–84.

O'Brien, Susan. 2001. Spirit discipline: Gender, Islam, and hierarchies of treatment in postcolonial Northern Nigeria. *Interventions* 3 (2): 222–41.

Ogala, William Nuhu. 1971. Beggars in Zaria. Long essay, Department of Community Medicine, Ahmadu Bello University, Zaria.

Okpani, Ikenna. 2003a. Anti-polio vaccine campaign unnecessary—Senator Tafida. *Daily Trust,* 20 November.

———. 2003b. FG declares polio vaccine safe. *Daily Trust,* 24 December.

Okunade, Adebimpe O. 1981. Attitude of Yoruba of Western Nigeria to handicap in children. *Childcare Health and Development* 7:187–94.

Olaniyi, Rasheed. 2006. Approaching the study of the Yorùbá Diaspora in Northern Nigeria. In *Yoruba Identity and Power Politics,* ed. T. Falola and A. Genova, 231–50. Rochester, N.Y.: University of Rochester Press.

Olatimehin, Oluwole. 1988. Accomplishing the goal of EPI. *National Concord,* 27 April.

Olayinka, Collins. 2007a. Immunisation body, primary healthcare agency for merger. *Guardian,* 8 May. http://www.guardiannewsngr.com, accessed 8 May 2009.

———. 2007b. Zamfara residents reject polio vaccines. *Guardian,* 29 January. http://www.guardiannewsngr.com, accessed 29 January 2009.

Oliver-Bever, Bep. 1986. *Medicinal Plants in Tropical West Africa.* Cambridge: Cambridge University Press.

Olusanya, Bola. 2004. Polio-vaccination boycott in Nigeria. *Lancet* 363 (9424): 1912.

Onwuejeogwu, Michael. 1969. The cult of the *bori* spirits among the Hausa. In *Man in Africa,* ed. M. Douglas and P. Kaberry, 279–305. London: Tavistock.

Orere, Onajomo. 1989. Minister pledges to meet immunisation target next year. *Guardian,* 13 December.

Oroye, Joe. 2005. Obasanjo urges Nigerians to improve children's health. *Daily Trust,* 10 August.

Oshinsky, David. 2005. *Polio: An American Story.* Oxford: Oxford University Press.

Outbreak of Smallpox. Vaccination Campaign Reports. 1955–57. KAD-MOH, file DIS 23, vol. 3, Nigerian National Archives, Kaduna.

Owens-Ibie, Nosa. 2005. Against the odds: Kano cripples take action to fight polio. http://www.who.int/countries/nga/features/2005/odds/en/index.html, accessed 14 November 2007.

Pallansch, Mark, and Hardeep Sandhu. 2006. The eradication of polio—progress and challenges. *New England Journal of Medicine* 355 (24): 2508–11.

Parry, Elydryd, R. Godfrey, D. Mabey, and G. Gill, eds. 2004. *Principles of Medicine in Africa.* Cambridge: Cambridge University Press.

Paul, John. 1971. *A History of Poliomyelitis.* New Haven, Conn.: Yale University Press.

Petryna, Adriana. 2005. Ethical variability: Drug development and globalizing clinical trials. *American Ethnologist* 32 (2): 183–97.

Pfeiffer, J. 2004. International NGOs in the Mozambique health sector: The "velvet glove" of privatization. In *Unhealthy Health Policy: A Critical Anthropological Examination,* ed. Arachu Castro and Merrill Singer, 43–62. Walnut Creek, Calif.: Altamira Press.

Pifer, John, and C. L. Adeoye. 1968. Characteristics of an epidemic of smallpox, Gerere Hamlet, Nigeria—1968. World Health Organization Library, file WHO/SE/68.5.

Polgreen, Lydia. 2005. Nigeria in deal to pay off most of its foreign debt. *New York Times,* 21 October.

Polio Information Center Online, Department of Microbiology and Immunology, Columbia University. 2002. Polio epidemiology. http://microbiology.columbia.edu/PICO/Chapters/Epidemiology.html, accessed 12 July 2009.

Poliomyelitis. 1947–57. KAD-MOH, file DIS 14, vol. 1, Nigerian National Archives, Kaduna.

Poliomyelitis Inoculation. 1957–59. KAD-MOH 1/18, Y199, Nigerian National Archives, Kaduna.

Rabiu, Ruby. 2007. FG files criminal charges against Pfizer. *Daily Trust,* 26 July.

———. 2008a. Bauchi: Polio immunization suffers set back. *Daily Trust,* 9 February.

———. 2008b. Six clerics stop polio immunization in Niger. *Daily Trust,* 28 July. http://www.dailytrust.com, accessed 28 July 2008.

———. 2009. Nigeria's low health indices blamed on corruption. *Daily Trust,* 12 June.

Rapp, Rayna, and Faye Ginsburg, eds. 2002. Disability. *Public Culture* 13:533–56.

Razum, Oliver, Onkar Mittal, Ritu Priya, K. R. Nayar, and C. Sathyamala. 2004. Language use in public health. *Lancet* 363 (9427): 2190–91.

Reeler, A. V. 2000. Anthropological perspectives on injections: A review. *Bulletin of the World Health Organization* 78 (1):135–43.

Rehabilitation of beggars. 1966–67. KADMINHEALTH 1/18, MOH file no. 5392, Nigerian National Archives, Kaduna.

Renne, Elisha. 1996. Perceptions of population policy, development, and family planning in Northern Nigeria. *Studies in Family Planning* 27 (3): 127–36.

———. 2006. Perspectives on polio and immunization in Northern Nigeria. *Social Science & Medicine* 63 (7): 1857–69.

———. 2009. Anthropological and public health perspectives on the polio eradication initiative in Northern Nigeria. In *Anthropology and Public Health: Bridging Differences in Culture and Society,* ed. R. Hahn and M. Inhorn, 512–38. New York: Oxford University Press.

Rey, Michaël, and Marc Girard. 2008. The global eradication of poliomyelitis: Progress and problems. *Comparative Immunology, Microbiology and Infectious Diseases* 31 (2–3): 317–25.

Reynolds, Toby. 2007. Polio: An end in sight. *British Medical Journal* 335:852–54.

Roberts, Leslie. 2006. Polio eradication: Is it time to give up? *Science* 312 (5775): 832–35.

———. 2007a. Polio: No cheap way out. *Science* 316 (5823): 362–63.

———. 2007b. Vaccine-related polio outbreak in Nigeria raises concerns. *Science* 317 (5846): 1842.

Rogers, Naomi. 1992. *Dirt and Disease: Polio before FDR.* New Brunswick, N.J.: Rutgers University Press.

Rosenberg, Charles. 1992. Framing disease: Illness, society, and history. Introduction to *Framing Disease: Studies in Cultural History,* ed. Charles E. Rosenberg and Janet Golden, xiii–xxvi. New Brunswick, N.J.: Rutgers University Press.

Sa'idu, Isa. 2008. Zaria: Water shortage threatens lives. *Weekly Trust,* 1 March.

Sa'idu, Isa, and Yusha'u Ibrahim. 2007. Special Report: Measles ravages Zaria City. *Sunday Trust,* 16 December. http://www.dailytrust.com, accessed 17 December 2007.

Salk Anti-poliomyelitis Vaccine. 1956–61. KAD-MOH 1/18, MH 5079, Nigerian National Archives, Kaduna.

Sam, Victor, and Francis Falola. 2008. Yar'Adua sacks national primary healthcare boss. *Punch,* 17 October. http:/h3.punchng.com, accessed 1 November 2008.

Samuelsen, Helle. 2001. Infusions of health: The popularity of vaccinations among Bissa in Burkina Faso. *Anthropology and Medicine* 8 (2–3): 164–75.

Sanghavi, Darshak. 2006. Wanting babies like themselves, some parents choose genetic defects. *New York Times,* 5 December.

Schimmer, Barbara, and Chikwe Ihekweazu. 2006. Polio eradication and measles immunisation in Nigeria. *Lancet Infectious Diseases* 6 (2): 63–65.

Schram, Ralph. 1971. *A History of the Nigerian Health Services.* Ibadan: University of Ibadan Press.

Scott, James. 1985. *Weapons of the Weak.* New Haven, Conn.: Yale University Press.

Shuaibu, Mohammed L. 2007. Handicapped boy calls for help. *Daily Trust,* 7 August.

Singh, Nishith K., Vineet Gupta, and Vikas K. Singh. 2007. Correspondence. *Lancet* 370 (9582): 132.

Smallpox eradication and measles control campaign. 1966–67. KADMINHEALTH 2/72, MOH file V.855, vol. 1, Nigerian National Archives, Kaduna.

Smith, Mary F. 1954. *Baba of Karo, a Woman of the Muslim Hausa.* New Haven, Conn.: Yale University Press.

Soares, Benjamin. 2005. *Islam and the Prayer Economy: History and Authority in a Malian Town*. Edinburgh: Edinburgh University Press (for the International African Institute).

Stephens, Joe. 2000. Where profits and lives hang in balance. *Washington Post*, 17 December.

———. 2006. Panel faults Pfizer in '96 clinical trial in Nigeria. *Washington Post*, 7 May.

Stones, P. B. 1961. The control of poliomyelitis. *West African Medical Journal* 10:222–26.

Sule, Bello. n.d. *Shan Inna*. A public service broadcast, narrated by Rafa'i Bawa Dalhatu. UNICEF-Bauchi Office and the Nigerian Television Authority.

Suleiman, Tajudeen. 2007. Ordeal of "drug" victims. *Tell* 31:48–51.

Sutter, Roland W., Vistor M. Cáceres, and Pedro Mas Lago. 2004. The role of routine polio immunization in the post-certification era. *Bulletin of the World Health Organization* 82 (1): 31–39.

Synge, Richard. 2001. *Africa South of the Sahara 2001*. 30th ed. London: Europa.

Taylor, Carl E., Felicity Cutts, and Mary E. Taylor. 1997. Ethical dilemmas in current planning for polio eradication. *American Journal of Public Health* 87 (6): 922–25.

Tayo, Adekunle. 1989. I don't want to beg for alms. *Sunday Sketch*, April 23.

Thompson, David, and William Foege. 1968. Faith Tabernacle smallpox epidemic, Abakaliki, Nigeria. World Health Organization Library, file WHO/SE/68.3.

Thompson, Kimberly M., and Radboud J. Duintjer Tebbens. 2007. Eradication vs. control for poliomyelitis: An economic analysis. *Lancet* 369 (9570): 1363–71.

Tomori, Oyewole. 2006. *Politics and Disease Control in Nigeria*. Ibadan: Archives of Ibadan Medicine.

Treamearne, Arthur J. N. 1914. *The Ban of the Bori: Demons and Demon-Dancing in West and North Africa*. London: Frank Cass, 1968.

Trevitt, Lorna. 1973. Attitudes and customs in childbirth amongst Hausa women in Zaria City. *Savannah* 2:223–26.

Ugwu, Emmanuel. 1996. UNICEF moves in. *Newswatch* 24 (6): 31.

Umar, Abubakar. 1989. No free EPI vaccines to states from '90. *New Nigerian*, 27 October.

Umar, Baffa A. 2006. *Child Immunisation: Muslim Reactions in Northern Nigeria*. Kano: International Institute of Islamic Thought.

Umar, Muhammad Sani. 1993. Changing Islamic identity in Nigeria from the 1960s to the 1980s: From Sufism to anti-Sufism. In *Muslim Identity and Social Change in Sub-Saharan Africa*, ed. L. Brenner, 154–78. Bloomington: Indiana University Press.

UNICEF (United Nations Children's Fund). 2009. *Immunization Summary: A Statistical Reference Containing Data through 2007*. New York: UNICEF; Geneva: World Health Organization.

USAID (United States Agency for International Development). 1994. USAID's strategy for stabilizing world and population growth and protecting human health. Memorandum 200. *Population and Development Review* 20 (2): 483–87.

———. 2006. Polio victims advocate for polio eradication. *U-Said-It Newsletter*, March. http://www.nigeria-usaidit.org/news/newsletter/mar2006/newsletter-mar2006 .php?story=polio, accessed 14 November 2007.

Vaccination Campaign Reports. 1949–1954. File 52, vol. 1, Nigerian National Archives, Kaduna.

van Staa, AnneLoes, and Anita. Hardon. 1996. *Injection Practices in the Developing World: A Comparative Review of Field Studies in Uganda and Indonesia*. Geneva: World Health Organization.

Veenman, Justus, and Lammert Jansman. 1980. The 1978 Dutch polio epidemic: A socio-logical study of the motives for accepting or refusing vaccination. *Netherlands Journal of Sociology* 16:21–48.

Walker, Andrew. 2007a. Nigerians try to dampen polio fears. *BBC News,* 16 October. http://news.bbc.co.uk/2/hi/africa/7046680.stm, accessed 16 October 2007.

———. 2007b. Polio immunization delayed in Kano. *Daily Trust,* 24 November. http://dailytrust.org/ accessed 27 November 2007.

Wall, Lewis. 1988. *Hausa Medicine.* Durham, N.C.: Duke University Press.

Washington Post 2009. Nigeria and Pfizer near deal on child deaths. *Washington Post,* 3 April. http://www.washingtonpost.com, accessed 7 April 2009.

Weekly Trust. 2003. "We will not submit our children for vaccination."—Emir of Kaza-ure. Conversation between Najeeb H. Adamu, emir of Kazaure, and Dr. Gloria Mugandu. 8–14 November.

Weiss, Holger. 2007. Begging and almsgiving in Ghana: Muslim positions towards pov-erty and distress. Research report No. 133. Uppsala: Nordiska Afrikainstitutet.

WHA. *See* World Health Assembly.

Whitting, C. E. 1940. *Hausa and Fulani Proverbs.* Lagos: Government Printer.

WHO. *See* World Health Organization.

Whyte, Susan R., and Sjaak van der Geest. 1994. Injections: Issues and methods for an-thropological research. In *Medicines: Meanings and Contexts,* ed. N. Etkin and M. L. Tan, 137–61. Quezon City: Health Action Information Network.

Wilks, Ivor. 1965. A note on the early spread of Islam in Dagomba. Transactions of the Historical Society of Ghana 8:87–98.

Wilson, Brenda. 2005. Health professionals in Kano, Nigeria, still have reservations about the Western-led polio immunization campaign. *Morning Edition,* NPR News, 13 April.

World Bank. 2008. Project paper on a proposed additional financing: Partnerships for Polio Eradication Project. Report no. 44776-NG. Abuja: World Bank, Africa Re-gion Office. http://www-wds.worldbank.org, accessed 1 November 2008.

World Health Assembly. 1988a. Global eradication of poliomyelitis by the year 2000: Plan of action. Geneva: World Health Organization. http://dosei.who.int/uhtbin/cgisirsi/NtROHT8mS5/19890032/5/0, accessed 21 May 2007.

———. 1988b. Global eradication of poliomyelitis by the year 2000. Resolution WHA 41.28. Geneva: WHO. http://www.wemos.nl/documents/WHA41.pdf, accessed 22 May 2007.

———. 2007. Poliomyelitis: Mechanism for management of potential risks to eradication. Report by the Secretariat, 12 April, WHA A60/11. http://www.who.int/gb/ebwha/pdf_files/WHA60/A60_11-en.pdf, accessed 22 May 2007.

World Health Organization. 1996a. Cerebrospinal meningitis in Africa. *Weekly Epide-miological Record* 71 (12): 89–90.

———. 1996b. Cerebrospinal meningitis, Nigeria. *Weekly Epidemiological Record* 71 (10): 80.

———. 2000. *Global Polio Eradication Initiative, Strategic Plan 2001–2005.* Geneva: WHO.

———. 2007a. Contributions and pledges to the Global Polio Eradication Initiative, 1985–2009. http://www.polioeradication.org/poliodonors.asp, accessed 26 October 2007.

———. 2007b. National immunization days and supplementary national immunization ac-tivities calendar, 2001–2007, Nigeria. http://www.who.int/immunization_monitoring/en/globalsummary/siacalendar/padvancedsia.cfm, accessed 26 October 2007.

————. 2007c. Polio vaccinations in Nigeria. A video diary of Immunization Plus Days, Nigeria, June 2007. http://www.polioeradication.org/videoaudio.asp, accessed 26 October 2007.

————. 2007d. Quarterly update. *Polio Lab Network* 13 (1): 1–4.

————. 2009. Polio case count. http://www.who.int/immunization_monitoring/en/diseases/poliomyelitis/case_count.cfm, accessed 11 December 2009.

World Health Organization, Ghana. 2003. A profile: Ghana's expanded programme on immunization in Ghana. Accra: Ghana Health Service. http://www.who.int/countries/gha/publications/EPI_Profile.pdf, accessed 21 June 2009.

World Health Organization, Kaduna. 2005. Kaduna State LGAs showing status of non compliance (NC), after August 2005 SNIDs. Unpublished printed summary.

————. 2006. Wild poliovirus cases, line list, Jan.–Aug. 2006. Unpublished.

————. 2007a. Immunization levels, Kaduna State, Jan.–June 2007. Unpublished.

————. 2007b. Wild poliovirus cases, line list, Jan.–Aug. 2007. Unpublished.

World Health Organization and UNICEF. 2007. Review of national immunization coverage, 1980–2006: Nigeria. http://www.who.int/immunization_monitoring/en/globalsummary/countryprofileselect.cfm, accessed 28 October 2007.

Wuaku Commission. 2002. Report: The Commission of Inquiry (Yendi Events). C.I. 36/2002. Tamale, Ghana: Tamale Institute of Cross-Cultural Studies Library.

Wyatt, H. V. 1984. The popularity of injections in the Third World: Origins and consequences for poliomyelitis. *Social Science & Medicine* 19 (9): 911–15.

————. 1992. Mothers, injections and poliomyelitis. *Social Science & Medicine* 35 (6): 795–98.

Yahya, Maryam. 2007. Polio vaccines—"no thank you!" Barriers to polio eradication in Northern Nigeria. *African Affairs* 106:185–204.

Yekutiel, P. 1980. *Eradication of Infectious Diseases: A Critical Study.* Basel: S. Karger.

Index

Burkina Faso: incidence of wild poliovius, 5, 86; National Immunization Days, 38; road network, 86, 96

"bush paths," 96, 98

Bwari Area Council, 77

Bwari School for Rehabilitating Beggars, 77, 78

census, 30; of the disabled, 83, 135n10

Centers for Disease Control and Prevention (CDC), 2, 5, 27, 45, 96, 109, 119, 136n5, 138n9

Cephtriaxone, 108

cerebrospinal meningitis, 15, 19, 31, 34, 107, 108, 119, 131n1

cerebrospinal meningitis epidemics: 1949–51, 129n12; 1996, 40, 48, 107

childhood diseases, 18, 25, 35, 36, 66. *See also* diphtheria; malaria; measles; pertussis; polio; tetanus; tuberculosis; vaccine-preventable childhood diseases

Children's Neurology Clinic, University College Hospital, Ibadan, 25

chloroquine, 59

Christians, 9, 10, 128nn13,14

cin zanzana (smallpox), 17, 19

circulating vaccine-derived poliovirus (cVDPV), 2, 8, 13, 103, 109–110, 112, 115, 120, 121, 122, 137nn6,7, 138n9, 139n15; 2005–2009 outbreak, 2, *3t,* 11, 134n18, 135n1. *See also* vaccine, oral polio

civilization (*zamani*), 30–31

Clapperton, Hugh, 20, 54, 128n1

Cohen, Abner, 70, 135n3

"cold legs" (*sanyi kafa*), 44

colonial government: in Ghana, 83; in Northern Nigeria, 21, 23, 105, 128n15

colonial health administration in Nigeria: health officers, 31; medical officers, 2, 25, 27, 31, 129n6, 133n9; medical service in North, 20, 21, 24, 105, 107

Colonial Office, 24

colonial railroad and road system in Northern Nigeria, 68–69

colonial officials: in Ghana, 68, 69, 129n9; in Nigeria, 21, 25, 71, 76, 131n14

community drama, 46, *plate 2*

Community Participation for Action in the Social Sector (COMPASS), 45–46, 48, 69; program, 83, 132n15

"cooling medicines," 19

Côte d'Ivoire: incidence of wild poliovius, 86; road network, 73, 86, 96

Cotonou, Republic of Benin, 96

Cuban Medical Brigade in Northern Region, Ghana, 94

cultural relativism, 102, 137n1

Dagomba, 87, 94, 136n8

dan Fodio, Abdullahi, 54, 56, 66

dan Fodio, Sheikh Usman, 52, 53, 54, 64, 66, 133n2

dar al-Islam, 15

debt relief, 92

Decree No. 12 of 1997, 37

Demographic and Health Surveys, Nigeria, 36, 133n12

Demonstration School for the Deaf, Kawa, Nigeria, 79

Denham, Dixon, 20

Department of Community Medicine, ABU, 16, 60

Department of Social Welfare and Community Development, colonial Ghana, 71

deworming medicine, 2, 44, 117

Dikwa, Borno State, 105–106

diphtheria-pertussis-tetanus (DPT-3) vaccine, 26, 35, 36, 44, 121, 131n8

disability: and stigma, 74, 81; categories of, 78; concepts of, 11–12, 68, 82, 83, 84; Hausas concept of, 68, 81, 134n1; reassessment of, 74, 78; strategies for overcoming, 12. *See also* beggars; begging; lame

disability rights, 69, 78; and development, 78, 85; education, 78; international initiatives, 78–79, 85; organizations, 78, 79; shift from self-help groups to government-funded groups

the disabled, 79; census of, 83; education, 79, 80, 82, 83; employment, 78, 84; federal programs, 81; in well-to-do families, 84; maintaining students in school, 79, 80; marriage, 135nn3,6; organizations, 78; Kaduna State programs, 78–81; self-help groups, 46, 71, 73–74, 78; vocational training, 79, 80, 83. *See also* beggars; the blind; the deaf; the lame (*guragu*); polio-disabled; and *names of specific organizations*

Disabled Business Association, Kaduna State, 78

"disease frames," 17, 18

"diseases of the affluent"; "diseases of the poor," 104

distrust: of American population policy, 65; of Nigerian government, 6, 30, 31, 34, 40, 41, 50, 63, 100; of private immunization by

Hadith, 10, 51, 53, 56, 66, 133nn2,10
Hassan, Alhaji Garba, 71, 73, 74, 75, 78, 96,
    plate 5
Hausa: concepts of disability, 68–69, 70;
    medical scholarship, 54–57; migrants, 73;
    migrants in Ghana, 71, 129n9, 135n2;
    migrants in Ibadan, 70, 135n3; proverbs and
    songs, 70; society, 7, 11, 12, 17, 84, 86, 95,
    135n11; trade network, 68–69, 86–87. *See
    also* mobile populations
Hausa medical specialists (*boka*): 23, 51, 59,
    62, 66, 81, 82, 89, 105; blood-letting
    and circumcision (*unwanzani*), 52;
    bone-setters (*mai dori*), 52, 59; herbalists
    (*mai magani*), 52
Hausa medicine (*magani gargarjiya*), 15, 18, 19,
    52, 54, 57; association with *bori,* 53; *turare*
    (medicinal smoke), 82; un-Islamic aspects,
    53; use of amulets, 17, 66, 128n3; use of
    herbal remedies, 17, 18, 23, 31, 55, 128n1; use
    of *rubutu,* 59. *See also* prayer
Hausa-Fulani, 9, 128n11, 128n13
health cards, 30, 44
health care equity, 103, 104, 106, 115
health incentives, 34, 42, 44, 48, 90, 101. *See
    also* bed nets; deworming medicine; measles
    vaccination; soap; Vitamin A supplements
health infrastructure, 13, 15, 31, 35, 88, 115, 116
health officials: international, 2, 17, 18; Native
    Authority, 26
health parastatals, Nigeria, 131n3
health workers in northeastern Ghana, 94;
    experience in National Immunization Days,
    92, 93, 99; problems of, 91, 136n9
health workers in Northern Nigeria, 106, 113,
    115, 117; colonial, 17; community, 83;
    complaints about, 48; experience in
    National Programme on Immunization, 43,
    44, 45; experience in Polio Eradication
    Initiative, 33, 38, 39, 40, 41, 43, 110, 130n20;
    experience in Smallpox Eradication
    Campaign, 30; impact of religious identity,
    86; impact of migration, 86; NGOs, 117;
    opposition to Polio Eradication Initiative,
    127n6; participation in strikes, 37; poor or
    inadequate training of, 58, 119, 121, 138n8;
    women, 130n20
health workers' strike, 96
hepatitis B, 58, 121, 131n8
herbal medicines, 17, 18, 23, 31, 52, 55, 128n1
"herd immunity." *See also* immunity
Heavily Indebted Poor Country Initiative, 92
HIV-AIDS, 9, 13, 15, 39, 49, 104

"hot" medicines, 19
Husseini, Malam, 55, 59–60, *plate 4*

Ibadan, 8, 25, 26, 70, 73, 129n7, 135n3
Idris, Alhaji Shehu, Emir of Zaria, 40, 63
immune system, 5, 51, 57, 134n16; American
    views of, 132n1
immunity: community, 13; "herd immunity,"
    13, 35, 104; *kariya Allah* (Hausa term for
    natural immunity), 51; natural immunity,
    19, 38; natural immunity to polio, 15, 25, 51,
    107, 127n1, 130n15; to polio, 5, 8, 13, 24,
    31–32, 35, 90, 104, 121
immunization in northeastern Ghana, 87–88;
    childhood, 89, 91; participation of Muslim
    community, 87
immunization in Nigeria, 3, 6: colonial era, 60;
    concepts of, 52; decline in routine
    childhood, 35; difficulties in implementa-
    tion, 127n7; failures of, 24; levels of, 5, 7, 8,
    13, 21, 33; low levels of routine immuniza-
    tion in Kaduna State, 48; low levels in Zaria
    Local Government, 60, 61, 62, 63; improve-
    ment in 2009, 2; mass events, 28; polio, 11,
    26, 31–32; protocols, 14; routine childhood,
    resistance to, 6, 20, 29, 44, 60, 91, 99, 100,
    126; services, 12; smallpox, 28–29, 32. *See
    also* vaccination
immunization team members, 15, 42, 43, 46,
    49, 63, 69, 95, 96, 113, 124, 127n7
Immunization Plus Days (2006), 33, 62, 67, 83,
    86, 101, 113, 120; addressing parents'
    concerns about primary health care, 2, 7, 14;
    community participation, 34, 46, 69;
    incentives, 117; improved provision of
    vaccines, 7; in Ghana, 86; organizational
    changes, 44, *plate 1*; political leaders'
    support, 63; success, 45, 47
infant and child mortality: in Ghana, 100;
    in Northern Nigeria, 100, 137n14
Infectious Disease Hospital, Kano, 108
infertility, 13, 60, 87, 100
infertility drugs, 9, 15
infrastructure, 7, 15, 23, 30, 31, 33, 88,
    115, 116
injection-therapy, 89
injections, 1, 9, 44, 51, 57, 58, 59, 60, 62, 122.
    association with needles, 57; distrust of, 42,
    60; fear of, 66; increasing paralysis, 59;
    ineffectual for spiritual disorders, 59–60;
    safety, 92, 100; source of healing, 89; source
    of infection, 51–52, 58, 62; source of
    paralysis, 58, 59, 60, 89, 132n9; source of

nerve damage, 59; interpretations in Yendi and Zaria, 89, 133n7. *See also allura*
Inter-Agency Coordinating Committee, Ghana, 92
International Fiqh Council, 63
International Monetary Fund (IMF), 35, 92, 105
International Red Cross, 26, 76, 83
Iran, 65
Islam, 10, 11, 15–16, 18, 23, 51–67; and health care reform, 55; and immunization, 68, 70, 74, 76, 84, 107, 113
Islamic education, 10, 12, 67, 132n11
Islamic medicine, 52–54, 55–57, 67
Islamic sects (Izala, Qadiriyya, Salafiyya, Shi'a, Sufi, Tijaniyya), 10. *See also* Izala, Sufi, Salafiya
Islamic texts, 10, 51, 55
Islamiyya schools, 10, 47, 56, 66, 67, 123
Islamiyya teachers, 48, 49, 56
Ilorin, Kwara State, 25, 28
Izala (Jama'atu Izalat al-Bid'a wa Iqamat al-Sunna), 10, 53, 54, 56, 128n12, 133n10, *plate 3*

Jama'atu Izalat al-Bid'a wa Iqamat al-Sunna. See Izala
Jama'atu Nasril Islam, 39, 40, 63, 130n22
James, William, 102
Jigawa State, 46, 120, 135n10
jihad (1804), 52, 53, 54, 55, 133n2
jinn. *See aljanu*
Joint National Association of Disabled People (JUNADP), 78
Jos, 25, 58, 76

Kadandani, 24
Kaduna State, 16, 40, 58, 69, 136n12; begging, 84; *bori* practices, 130n14; cerebrospinal meningitis, 131n1; confirmed polio cases, 8, 45; development, 125, 126; measles fatalities, 61; polio campaigns, 39, 46; primary health care, 48; programs for the disabled, 73, 74, 76, 78–79, 83; smallpox eradication campaign, *27*, 129n9; unemployment, 30; vaccination centers, 27, WHO video, 127n7. *See also* immunization; *individual entries for Kaduna State government institutions*
Kaduna State Ministry of Education Scholarship Board, 80
Kaduna State Ministry of Health, 61
Kaduna State National Programme on Immunization, 16

Kaduna State Office for Special Education, Ministry of Education, 79, 80–81
Kaduna State Rehabilitation Board, 79
Kaduna State Rehabilitation Centre, 79–80
Kaduna State Rehabilitation Centre Board (RCB), 79
Kaduna State Special Education School, 79, 80
Kafanchan, 25
Kano (city), 7, 28, 39, 80, 95, 136n10; railroad, 73. *See also* Baba of Karo; begging; COMPASS; the disabled; Immunization Days Plus; Kano State polio boycott; Kano State Polio Victims Trust Association; Musa Muhammad; paralysis; Pfizer Trovan drug trial; polio; Polio Eradication Initiative; traditional healers; vaccine-derived poliovirus; vaccines for polio
Kano Polio Victims Trust Association, 83
Kano State, 39, 40, 83, 84, 107, 108, 112, 128n10, 138n12
Kano State polio immunization boycott, 2, 64, 98, 131n5
kariya Allah (natural immunity). *See* immunity
kashin (feces), 19
Katsina State, 25, 46, 63, 73, 128n2
Kebbi State, 46, 96, 123
Kennedy, President John F., 65
"Kick Polio Out of Africa" slogan, 113
Kofar Gayan State Hospital, 81
Koleoso-Adelekan, Titilola, 48
Konkomba, 94, 95, 136n8
Kpunkpano village (Yendi District), 89
kungiyar guragu (association of the lame), 71, 73, 74, 80, 135n4
Kungiyar Guragu Zazzau, 73–74

Laboratory Service, Yaba, Lagos, 22
Lagos, 7, 24, 25, 28, 71, 73, 96; smallpox cases, 129n10
Lambo, Eyitayo, 9, 39
lame (*gbalibila fiep-fiep,* Dagbani) in northeastern Ghana, 87, 99
lame (*gurgu* [m.], *gurguwa* [f.], *guragu* [pl.], Hausa), in Northern Nigeria: 11, 68; access to education, 67, 69; associations of, 71–74, 78; *bori* spirit, 31; causes, 84; girls, 128n16; Hausa concept and definition, 69–70; difficulties in Hausa society, 12; marriage of, 75; men, 11, 68; occupations of, 71, 83, 84; Qur'anic teaching about, 70; vocational training, 83; women, 23, 75. *See also* beggars; disabilities; the disabled

"normal life" (*zaman daidai*), 69

Northern Nigeria, 3, 5, 7; colonial era, 2, 20, 21, 23, 24, 25, 27, 31, 71, 76, 105, 107, 128n15, 131n14, 133n9; connection with northern Ghana, 135n2; education system, 10, 43, 78, 79, 83, 84, 91; epidemics, 19, 20, 21, 64, 107, 109, 110, 129n12; health policy, 42, 55, 81; historical influence of Islam, 10, 15, 52; independence, 29; infant mortality rate, 137n14; Islamic law, 131n6; map of migrant route to Ghana, 72; Muslim identity in, 10, 31; political instability, 52, 91; pre-Islamic religious practices, 18, 20, 23; road networks, 86, 96, 97. *See also* comparison with Northeastern Ghana; the disabled,; National Expanded Programme on Immunisation; National Immunization Days; Polio Eradication Initiative

The North, Republic or Monarchy? (Sa'adu Zungur), 84

Northeastern Ghana, 86, 87; origins of Islam, 135n2; transnational ethnic groups, 95. *See also* Polio Eradication Initiative; wild poliovirus

Northern Province, Nigeria, 20, 21, 76

Northern Region, Ghana, 91; comparison to Northern Nigeria, 99–100, 135n3; ethnic conflict, 94–95, 100; guinea worm eradication, 136n7; impact of 2003–2004 Kano polio vaccination boycott, 98; roads, 97; scarcity of health services, 94; transnational ethnic groups, 95, 99; under-five mortality rate, 136n13. *See also* Ghanaian Expanded Programme on Immunisation; health workers; Polio Eradication Initiative; polio immunization

Nuhu Bamalli Polytechnic, 82

Obasanjo, President Olusegun, 9, 41, 48, 112, 116

Office of Social Welfare, Ministry of Health, Nigeria, 128n15

Olobiri town, Niger Delta, 130n18

"one right against another right" (Das), 106

ordinary people (*talakawa*), 64

Osotimehin, Babatunde, 48

Panadol, 15

paracetamol, 15, 48, 90

paralysis, 2, 5, 8, 9, 11–12, 18, 23, 25, 44, 53, 58–59, 84, 99, 121, 133n3; acute flaccid paralysis, 2, 3t, 8, 11, 23, 33, 37–38, 83, 105, 120, 138n9; association with *bori* spirits, 11,

31, 59, 70, 89, 90, 129n13; association with vaccine, 88, 110, 132n9; causes, 2, 89

Paralyze (style of dress), 128n18

Pate, Muhammed Ali, 48

Ped-O-Jet injector, 27

pertussis vaccine, 35

Pfizer, Inc., 107–108, 137n4

Pfizer Trovan drug trial, 107–109; *Daily Trust* publication of hearing, 137n5; *Washington Post* stories, 108. *See also* Abdullahi vs. *Pfizer, Inc.* (2005)

Physically Handicapped Association of Nigeria (PHAN), 78, 80

polio: definition, 16; epidemics in U. S., 5, 15; increase of expatriate cases in colonial Nigeria, 24; monitoring in independent Nigeria, 37, 138n9; monitoring system in colonial Nigeria, 32; traditional Northern Nigerian treatment, 23. *See also* poliomyelitis

the polio-disabled, 83; changing perspectives, 84; education, 69, 83; employment, 69; employment as beggars, 75, 85; informants, 71; marriage prospects, 75; microcredit facilities, 83; programs, 69, 84. *See also* beggars; begging; Community Participation for Action in the Social Sector (COMPASS)

polio eradication, 14, 15, 34, 50, 59, 63; argument against, 122–123; ethics of 101, 106

polio eradication campaigns, 14, 17, 30, 31, 32, 35; advertisement in Ghana, 93; in northeastern Ghana, 91, 95; in Northern Nigeria, 2, 3, 5, 7, 8, 9, 11, 18, 25, 41, 100; national strategy, 85, 91; worldwide efforts, 14, 38, 43, 46

Polio Eradication Initiative, Northeastern Ghana, 3, 86, 87; comparison with Northern Nigerian initiative, 87–88; government commitment, 87; spread of polio from Northern Nigeria, 86, success, 86

Polio Eradication Initiative, Northern Nigeria (1998–mid-2009), 2, 7, 15, 18, 29, 32, 60, 96, 103, 122, 126; acceptance, 98; comparison to Northeastern Ghana response, 86–90, 91, 100, 101; comparison to US measles eradication campaign, 119–120; cultural context, 87; ethical questions, 109–110; government commitment, 87; immunization boycott (2003–2004), 2; political context, 9, 16, 30, 33, 52; implementation, 34–39, 63–64, 67, 131n5; as priority in national primary health care

Polio Eradication Initiative (*continued*)
policy, 34, 105, 106, 112, 115–118; programs for disabled, 83; publicity, 33, radio and television publicity, 98, 113; reorganization, 43–59; resistance to, ix, 2, 7, 12, 13, 14, 16, 39, 45, 46, 49, 51, 52, 57, 60, 61, 63, 87, 91, 103, 109, 118, 120, 126, 134n18; Rotary International sponsorship, 6; socioeconomic context, 87, 115, 128n17; supporters, 3, 30, 34, 40, 63, 64, 67, 69; timeframe, 112; World Health Organization participation, 16; in Zaria, 40–43, 126. *See also* CDC; Rotary International; World Health Organization
"polio fatigue," 126
poliomyelitis, 1, 110, 112, 130n16; bori associations, 23, 31; cases in Adamawa State, 42; cases in Northern Nigeria, 47; causes, 5, colonial policy, 18, 22; colonial treatment, 24–26; diagnosis, 8, 11; epidemiology, 24, 34, 130n16; publicity (dress, radio, television), 40; symptoms, 2; transmission, 7, 24. *See also* polio; polio eradication; polio eradication campaigns; Polio Eradication Initiative; Northeastern Ghana; Polio Eradication Initiative, Northern Nigeria; polio vaccine. *See also* ethics
polio vaccine, 26, 29; contamination, 6, 9, 11, 15, 39, 41, 49, 56
Polio Victims Trust Association, 46, 67, 69, 83
politics, 9–11, 33, 35, 40, 52, 63–67, 122
political conflict, 36–37
popular culture, 16, 70, 116
prayer, 18, 51, 52, 53, 54, 55, 56, 59, 66
primary health care, in Islamic countries, 134n20
primary health care in Nigeria, 2, 7, 13, 35, 41, 42, 49, 87, 103, 117, 123, 126, 128n17, 131n2; comparison to Ghana, 100–101; decline, 3, 8, 12, 15, 40, 116; facilities, 35, 36, 120; in Zaria, 61; programs, 14, 36 48, 66, 88, 105, 106, 115–116; shift from federally operated system to local government operated, 105. *See also* Polio Eradication Initiative
primary health care in United Kingdom, 104
The Prophetic Medicine, 51, 52, 54
public health, 111; campaigns, 11, 13; initiatives, 13, 49–50, 103, 104, 114, 117; interventions, 83, 103, 104, 107; meaning, 11; policy, 13, 49, 83, 103, 105, 106; priorities, 18, 103, 105, 106; programs, 49, 50, 81, 104, 118; national campaigns, 46, 104; views, 6, 18, 102, 103

public health ethics, 103–105, 107, 110, 114; of eradication, 101, 103
public health organizations, international, 6, 34; national, 34. *See also* Centers for Disease Control and Prevention (CDC); Gates Foundation, International Red Cross; UNICEF; World Health Organization (WHO)
public health professionals, 13, 33, 42, 102, 103, 104, 111, 113, 114, 117; in Kano, 128n10; international, 2, 13, 17, 18, 21, 116; national, 2, 13, 21, 120; Northern Nigerian, 102; Western-trained, 18

Qir'a al-Ahibba, 54
Qu'ran, 19, 51, 55, 57, 66, 68, 102, 132, 133n10; on the disabled, 70; and gender mores, 15; and illness, 53, 56; and Muslim identity, 10; role in Northern Nigerian education, 10; use in making amulets, 18, 59, 66, 128n3

railroads, 68, 73
Rainbow Nursery and Primary School, Hotoro, Kano, 83
Ransome-Kuti, Olikoye, 35, 36
Red Cross. *See* International Red Cross
risk, 8, 57, 105, 115, 131n11; associated with vaccines, 6, 8, 9, 12, 42. 51, 52, 57, 103; of disease, 20, 51, 52, 122, 130n15; of paralysis, 6, 58, 121
road networks, 86, 95, 97; in northeastern Ghana, 96; in Nigeria, 7, 28, 32
Rotary International, 5, 13, 14, 20, 33, 34, 35, 37, 42 (immunization project), 83, 135n9; "no more rotary" graffiti, 6
routine immunization, 26, costs, 121; disruptions in Nigeria, 100, 101; effectiveness, 86, 122; in Ghana, 86, 87, 90, 91, 92, 93, 94, 99; impact of coercion, 107; impact of transnational movements, 99, 100; in Nigeria, 3, 35, 36, 37, 48, 51, 57, 60, 67, 115, 117, 120, 133n11; role in primary health care policy, 122, 126; resistance to, 61, 87; validity of WHO data, 110
rukiyya (exorcism), 19, 52
rumors, 3, 110; about contamination of Western commodities, 15; compared with 18th century Chinese rumors, 15; about HIV-AIDS and infertility, 13, 15, 39, 47, 49; in Ghana, 87; about safety of oral polio vaccine, 49, 109;

Elisha P. Renne is Professor in the Department of Anthropology and the Center for Afroamerican and African Studies at the University of Michigan–Ann Arbor. Her research focuses on the anthropology of health and development; gender relations; and religion and textiles, specifically in Nigeria. Her publications include *Population and Progress in a Yoruba Town; Regulating Menstruation* (edited with E. van de Walle); and *Cloth That Does Not Die,* as well as articles in *Africa, American Anthropologist, Journal of the Royal Anthropological Institute, Population and Development Review,* and *Social Science & Medicine.*